Silent Sufferers: Investigating Respiratory Illness Among Malawi's Tobacco Farmers

Shivani

Table of Contents

CHAPTER 1: INTRODUCTION AND LITERATURE REVIEW

1.1 INTRODUCTION AND BACKGROUND

Malawi has a population of about 17 million people. Most of the economically active are employed in the informal sector where 89% of the labor force is absorbed. Malawi's economy is known to heavily depend on agriculture for both subsistence and commercial reasons. Tobacco is the main cash crop [1] and Malawi is ranked among the five largest tobacco producers globally [2], relying on it as a major source of foreign revenue and involving about 20% of the national labor force. Tobacco cultivation in Malawi involves a considerable proportion of the labor force in all regions across the country. Farmers cultivate either as households or tenants as well as through employment in large estates. Most estates in the southern part of Malawi employ perennial casual labor on their estates.

The process of cultivating tobacco involves the use of chemicals, frequent contact with the tobacco leaves, and other exposures related to field preparation and tobacco processing such as curing. Given the magnitude of the population subjected to tobacco farm exposures in Malawi it is of paramount importance to understand the burden of tobacco related health effects in this particular population.

Studies have demonstrated that tobacco farm exposures are associated with diverse health effects including Green Tobacco Sickness (GTS) due to nicotine exposure, pesticide poisoning and respiratory disease as a result of skin and inhalational exposure[3]. A study by Plan International among Malawian tobacco farms focused on child labor revealed occurrence of green tobacco sickness in children but did not report on respiratory effects[4]. There is no documented study in this population to our knowledge that focused on the respiratory effects associated with tobacco cultivation. Several studies have been documented in Malawi concerning respiratory diseases in the general population but the majority have dwelled on infectious diseases[5]. Other studies that have investigated obstructive lung diseases are available but have not demonstrated the impact of workplace environment in such conditions[5,6].

Globally there is limited information about the role of tobacco farming in obstructive lung diseases such as Chronic Obstructive Pulmonary Disease (COPD) and asthma. The context in Malawi provides an opportunity to study and understand the relationship between tobacco farming exposures and prevalence of obstructive lung disease.

1.2 LITERATURE REVIEW

1.2.1 Literature search strategy

This review focusses on chronic respiratory diseases associated with tobacco cultivation with special attention to asthma and COPD. To identify relevant articles, a search was conducted on MEDLINE and Google scholar on respiratory health effects associated with tobacco farming within a period from 1970-2016 using different combinations of the following key words "tobacco farming" "respiratory health effects" "COPD" "asthma" "allergy" "nicotine farm exposure" "pesticides health effects" "organophosphates health effects" "HIV in farmers". These articles were further surveyed for additional citations, which were incorporated in the review if relevant. The review focused on characterizing tobacco farming and its associated exposures, exploring the common health effects reported by tobacco farmers and specifically focusing on articles dealing with chronic lung disease prevalent in this population. An evaluation of risk factors and potential confounders associated with obstructive lung disease in this population was also undertaken.

1.2.2 The tobacco cultivation process

Tobacco cultivation has shifted from high income countries (HICs) to low- and middle-income countries (LMICs) following campaigns against its cultivation in developed countries[7]. The negative health impacts of this shift are accentuated in the LMICs due to the lack of occupational health regulation, poverty as well as poor access to healthcare[8]. Among the top world tobacco producers are countries such as the United States of America, China, Brazil, India, and Malawi [1]. Malawi is unique in that it is heavily dependent on the crop for its economy as well as being the lowest income country listed among the significant tobacco producers. Due to the economic status of Malawi there is insufficient infrastructure to support such large- scale tobacco production and the use of modern farming technology is limited. This results in excessive manual work with indigenous and rudimentary methods of cultivation being employed in tobacco-farming. The larger quantity of tobacco produced in Malawi employs the use of sharecroppers[1,3] . These are contract farmers given land to farm. Sharecroppers are supplied with farm inputs with an agreement to share the produce with the land owners. This practice has been associated with the labour force being drawn from households in efforts to increase the share of small-scale farmers. According to the Food and Agriculture Organization (FAO), households' involvement in tobacco farming have been associated with a number of issues such as more people per household being exposed to adverse health effects and the use of child labour.

Malawi produces three main types of tobacco: Burley which forms about 82% (can reach 89%) of total mass production, followed by flue cured which constitutes about 17%, and dark-fired tobacco [9]. Burley is a light air cured variety that is mainly used for cigarette production and mainly produced by small holder famers who own their own small farms or as sharecroppers. The flue cured variety is produced by high earning large scale production estates which use casual and seasonal laborers for cultivation. Flue cured tobacco is dried in a closed building with furnace driven heat directed from flues that extend from the furnace into the barn. The dark-fired variety is dried by using wood smoke from small fires built on the floors of enclosed curing barns which gives it a characteristic flavor for chewing, snuff and pipe tobacco mixtures.

In Malawi, the tobacco season commences around July with preparation of nurseries and preparing beds for seeding. This involves tilling and hoeing mainly using hand held tools. After bed preparations, the beds are sterilized using chemicals or burning the top soil using dried biomass. Sowing follows this, and soon after sowing there is a judicious application of chemicals (pesticides and herbicides) in the nurseries to control different types of pests and weeds until transplantation time, which occurs after about 12 weeks. Following transplantation, the plants mainly grow by seasonal rains. During this phase, weeding as well as pest control occurs. Later, budding is controlled either chemically, or mechanically by removing them off the plant to improve leaf quality. This process occurs while the plant is at an advanced height and is associated with high exposure to nicotine from the buds and leaves especially when personal protective equipment is not worn. An outline of the various steps involved in tobacco cultivation is provided (Figure 1.1).

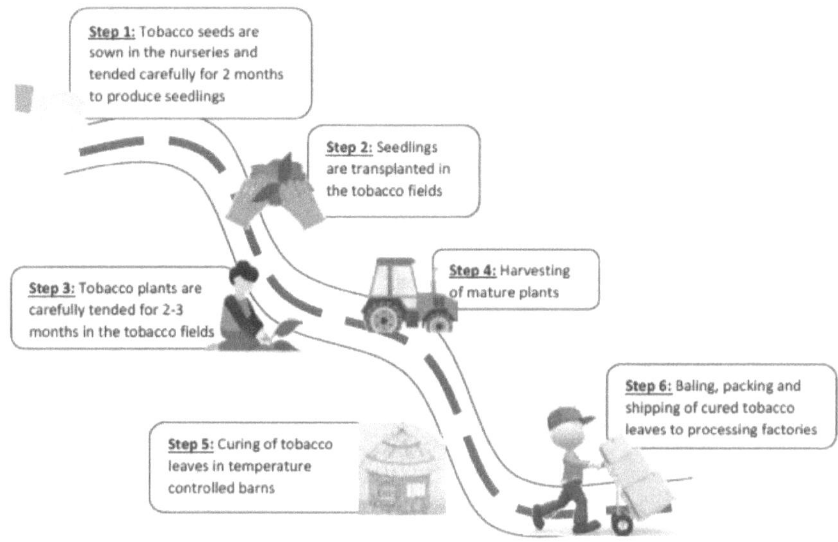

Figure 1.1: The typical tobacco cultivation process (with permission [8])

Pesticides in the Malawian context are applied by the sharecroppers as part of the whole cultivation process. As a monocrop, tobacco plants are vulnerable to a variety of pests and diseases, which require the application of large quantities of chemicals.[10] These include pesticides (insecticides, herbicides, fungicides and fumigants) and growth regulators (growth inhibitors and ripening agents), which are applied to the tobacco plants during different stages of growth.[10] In LMICs, pesticide and growth inhibitors are usually applied with hand held or backpack sprayers, without the use of the necessary protective equipment.[10] In Malawi the most widely used pesticides are neonicotinoids, organophosphates, and carbamates according to the Tobacco Control Commission. Some weeks after topping, harvesting occurs. Depending on the variety of tobacco, harvesting may occur in several rounds or once off. When it occurs once off tobacco is harvested by cutting the whole plant and taking off the leaves for stacking, later. In contrast, when harvesting in rounds only matured leaves are harvested, leaving behind the rest of the plant for the next round of harvest.

After harvesting the leaves are stacked into barns for drying in case of air drying for barley, or they are taken into curing barns for flue-cured or dark-fired varieties of tobacco. Except for air curing the other types of curing require the use of firewood smoke to give it a characteristic flavor. After drying the leaves are packed into bales for trading at an auction. Since the responsibility of cultivation is handled by households, although under the control of the Tobacco Commission of Malawi, the use of personal protection is suboptimal. Most of the farmers do not use protective equipment for protection against various hazards as these are perceived as additional costs of production and may be unaffordable. Some large estates that use casual labor as opposed to sharecroppers are responsible for providing personal protective equipment, however, there are no clear guidelines or regulation for safe handling of chemicals and tobacco plants made available to the employees.

1.2.3 Common occupational and environmental exposures associated with tobacco farming

Tobacco cultivation is associated with exposure to various hazards as a result of working in dusty environments, inhaling smoke when curing the tobacco, using chemicals such as pesticides during cultivation and nicotine from skin contact while harvesting the tobacco leaves (Table 1.1). The use of casual laborers in large estates exposes a very large group of employees to particular hazards. While it is expected that these estates should have capacity to supply and enforce PPE use among their employees, observation shows that this is not the case and it is not uncommon for these seasonal workers to forget some safety practices regarding their work in relation to prevailing hazards.

Table 1.1: Exposures associated with tobacco cultivation tasks

TASK	ACTIVITIES INVOLVED	POSSIBLE HAZARDS
Tilling	Use of hoes to break the soil to prepare beds	Organic and inorganic dust Sun Heat Ergonomic
Sterilizing the nursery	Rubble and straw are burnt on top of the prepared beds	Smoke from burning matter Heat
Chemical spraying	Use of sprayers and watering canes to mix, spray, then clean the equipment	Dermal, respiratory exposure to Pesticides and dermal exposure to Nicotine Ergonomic
Topping	Removal of the budding appendages	Dermal exposure to Nicotine Pesticides Ergonomic
Harvesting	Removal of the whole plant or leaves depending on the tobacco variety	Dermal exposure to Nicotine Ergonomic
Stacking	Systematically attaching and suspending the leaves for drying	Dermal exposure to Nicotine Ergonomic
Curing	Use of some form of fuels (e.g. wood) to generate heat for drying tobacco	Smoke from fuel combustion, Heat
Packing into bales	Sorting the leaves and packaging	Organic dust from leaves, mites, Ergonomic

1.2.3.1 Dose response relationships between exposures and their effects

Dust, nicotine and pesticides mediate their health effects in a dose dependent manner. Although nicotine effects tend to wane off with continued exposure due to tolerance, pesticides and dust effects worsen with continued and intensity of exposure [11].

Not much is known about the interaction of nicotine and pesticides at the pathophysiological level. A Thai study aimed at identifying correlation of health effects of nicotine and pesticides exposure, found that certain symptoms of GTS such as nausea and vomiting occurred at safe exposure levels to organophosphates, while headache and increased salivation were associated with higher exposure levels [12]. Wheezing was associated with having GTS in the previous year and those with more than 5 episodes in the previous year had twice the risk of developing wheezes according to a Brazilian study[13]. The limitation of this study is that no quantitative exposure measures were taken; either for nicotine or pesticides and it is difficult to determine whether this relationship had to do with retention of high nicotine levels in the body during the current year.

Several studies have demonstrated dose dependent health effects related to dust exposure among tobacco factory workers. Workers with a higher cumulative dust exposure had significantly lower lung indices against their predicted values compared to controls[14,15,16.]

Since tobacco cultivation involves concurrent exposure to dust as well as other chemicals such as pesticides and nicotine there is a need to evaluate their long-term respiratory effects among farmers.

1.2.3.1.1 Particulate tobacco Dust

Dust is defined as solid particles made airborne by the mechanical disintegration of bulk solid material or biological particles and usually consists of particles in sizes ranging from

1-100μm although ultrafine particles (UFPs) are usually less than 0.1μm. It is classified as inhalable, thoracic and respirable dust based on particle size. Inhalable dust (10 -100.0μm) is the fraction of total airborne particles that are inhaled through the nose and/or mouth. Thoracic dust (4-10μm) is that which can penetrate the respiratory system beyond the larynx. Respirable dust (4μm and below) is the fraction of airborne particles that can reach the alveoli where gas exchange occurs[17].

A Chinese study on tobacco dust exposure characterized the tobacco dust in a tobacco processing factory[15]. The average dust concentration ranged from 12.78 to 23.85mg/m^3. This was beyond the recommended average of vegetable dusts of 3mg/m^3. While most of the dust was organic the tobacco carried along other inorganic dust from the farms such as silica reaching close to 11% of the total dust content in tobacco. In this particular study between 80-97% of the measured particles were respirable dust.

Unlike the tobacco processing factory environment, cultivation is associated with exposure to both organic and inorganic dusts to a greater extent. The source of organic dust is the plant matter such as the dried tobacco leaves which is common in the barns and shades [13]. During field work workers are mainly exposed to inorganic dust from field soils which are usually composed of silica. A study in Zimbabwe among tobacco farmers reported levels of respirable tobacco dust of 19.13 ± 10.82 mg/m^3, which was much higher than the occupational exposure limit for inhalable dust[8].

There are no conventional occupational exposure limits for most dust encountered in tobacco farming. What is clear is that exposure to a mixture of organic and inorganic dusts makes it a complex exposure to quantify and assess. In China tobacco dust is grouped among vegetable dust and given an exposure limit of 3mg/m^3 for the processing factories[15]. Studies on tobacco farms of particulate dust levels report levels between 2-20mg/m^3 with some studies reporting levels as high as 100mg/m^3 among open cabin farm tractor drivers [18,19]. Several studies aimed at quantifying respirable dust levels using personal sampling among harvesters, showed concentrations of 0.52 to 2.16mg/m^3 while levels outside tractors were between 1.77 to 5.24 mg/m3 during field preparation[19]. A study among seasonal and permanent tobacco factory workers in Greece investigated suspended dust levels in a tobacco factory using static samples and showed concentrations of magnitude as high as 45.3 to 54.4 mg/m^3 [20]. This shows how dust is prevalent both in the tobacco fields as well as tobacco processing settings thereby posing some risk to workers in those environments.

Several factors have been demonstrated to be associated with changing dust particulate exposures in the field, which include differences in equipment, tasks, and climate. In one study, the presence of an enclosed tractor cabin, higher relative humidity, and lower tractor speed were both associated with lower dust exposure levels[19].

1.2.3.1.2 Nicotine

Nicotine is a water soluble odorless chemical and one of the chemicals produced by the tobacco plant. It has stimulatory effects on the central nervous and autonomic system through special *nicotinic* receptors [21]. It has tolerant and addictive effects on those exposed to it and its effects may not be appreciated even in higher doses in those chronically exposed to it. Nicotine can enter the body through dermal, oral, or by inhalation exposures. It is metabolized by the liver and excreted by the kidneys. Unlike the oral route, dermal and inhalation routes of exposures allow nicotine to reach the brain, lungs, and other organs without the first pass effect [21,22].

Most farmers are exposed to nicotine through dermal exposure involving contact with tobacco plants in the field during budding or harvesting. This poses a particular risk of high circulatory levels of nicotine especially during wet conditions [2]. Factors associated with high nicotine exposure include wet conditions, type of tobacco (Burley or Virginia tobacco have a high nicotine content and burley is predominant in Malawi), and alcohol consumption during work in tobacco cultivation and /or processing. Work practices such as longer work shifts, topping, and harvesting [2,3,7] all predispose to excessive nicotine exposure.

Nicotine is metabolized faster than most of its metabolites such as cotinine. Seventy percent of nicotine is extracted from the blood with each pass through the liver at a clearance rate of 1200ml per min compared to cotinine at 45ml per min. Because of its short half-life most studies have used metabolites such as cotinine for biological monitoring of nicotine exposure. Non-smoking status is generally associated with having a serum cotinine of less than 10ng/ml [23]. One study found cotinine levels of more than 10ng/ml among exposed tobacco workers [7]. Observed levels of cotinine above 50ng/ml/m^2 were associated with additional eye symptoms in exposed tobacco farmers [24].

A toxicological test on a patient with green tobacco sickness in Poland found cotinine levels as high as 869ng/ml [25]. One review demonstrated high cotinine levels in non-smoking tobacco farmers that were as high and comparable to smokers [2]. Not many toxicological studies have been published on quantitative analysis of nicotine exposure among tobacco farmers. Studies among tobacco farmers have instead focused on the use of symptomatology of nicotine related conditions such as green tobacco sickness to characterize its toxicity. This approach, however, has the potential to miss out exposure data among asymptomatic or tolerant individuals who might be harmed despite not manifesting with green tobacco sickness.

1.2.3.1.3 Pesticides

Pesticides are chemicals used to control diseases and parasites including weeds in agricultural production. Tobacco farming involves the utilization of a large amount of diverse pesticides. The application of these chemicals occurs at the beginning of the season and tapers down at different stages until harvesting which potentially results in continued chemical exposure to farmers. The common chemicals used in this regard are summarized in the Table 1.2 below.

The commonly used chemicals are organophosphates, pyrethroids, synthetic pyrethroids, and neonicotinoids, among others[26]. A study among Pakistani tobacco farmers reported a high concentration of neonicotinoid, carbamate, pyrethroid and organochlorine pesticide residues above the acceptable daily intake (ADI) for humans in the blood of tobacco farmers[8]. Health effects among pesticide handlers are associated with the type of pesticide, number of chemicals handled, use of protective equipment, duration of exposure/tasks, age, and gender.

Pesticide exposure occurs mainly through dermal, inhalation, and ingestion routes [27,28]. This allows the chemicals to reach the lungs without a first pass effect thereby exerting their possible effects before they are eliminated or altered. Most organophosphates are applied within two weeks after transplantation of seedlings is done. From transplantation to harvesting it takes about eight weeks. Most exposure to organophosphates occur during application which involves mixing, spraying, and cleaning of the instruments [29]. Although sprayers are the ones most at risk, any other farm workers in contact with the crop some days after spraying may also be exposed.

Different techniques have been used to monitor workers' exposure levels to organophosphates to address the issue of individual variations in dose response relationship. For organophosphates, a 50% reduction in Cholinesterase (ChE) from the baseline is associated with acute cholinergic or toxic symptoms and the recommended removal threshold for workers from exposure is a reduction of 60% for red cell ChE and 50% for plasma ChE. Workers may return to work if their ChE levels reach 75% of the baseline level [27,29]. However, chronic health effects related to organophosphates have been observed in individuals without necessarily showing significant difference of ChE levels compared to baseline [27].

Farmers are usually exposed to more than a single type of pesticide per growing season and the interaction between these combined effects are not well understood. Older age and female gender increase the risk of adverse effects [30].

Table 1.2: Pesticides used commonly in Malawi tobacco industry and reported associated respiratory effects among farming populations

Name of Group	Active Chemical	Associated Respiratory effect (Reference)
Neonicotinoids	Imidacloprid Acetamiprid Thiamethoxam	Respiratory irritation Reduced lung volumes (29)
Pyrethroids	Beta-cyfluthrin Deltamethrin Cyhalothrin	Wheeze, rhinitis, atopic, non-atopic asthma Chronic bronchitis (26,27,28)
Organophosphates	Dimethoate Chloropyriphos	Rhinitis, wheeze, reduced FEV1, atopic and non-atopic asthma Chronic bronchitis (26,27,28)
Herbicides	Trifulalin S Metolachlor	Rhinitis, wheeze, allergic asthma Chronic bronchitis (26,27,28)

1.2.4 Health effects associated with tobacco cultivation

1.2.4.1 Green Tobacco Sickness

Acute nicotine exposure in tobacco farmers has been associated with a condition called Green Tobacco Sickness (GTS). It occurs within hours of heavy exposure to nicotine and is usually self-limiting with spontaneous recovery in the next 48 hours [21]. It was first described in the 1970's as a neurotoxic syndrome characterized by headache, nausea, vomiting and headache. Other symptoms may also be present such as abdominal cramps, diarrhea and palpitations. It occurs as a result of stimulation of cholinergic receptors in the nervous system [3,21]. This is the most commonly documented specific health effect among tobacco farmers having a seasonal prevalence of up to 89% [2]. Incidence of GTS was shown to increase with time during the tobacco season [31]. It is more prevalent among young workers who are new to the occupation and those that come in contact with green tobacco leaves such as harvesters and chemical sprayers especially under wet conditions [32,33].

Hygiene measures such as hand washing and use of personal protective equipment, especially gloves, were associated with significant reduction in GTS in two separate studies [34,35]. Two interventional studies found a significant reduction (62-75%) of risk of GTS when rubber gloves were used compared with cotton gloves [35].

In a Brazilian study assessing prevalence of wheezing, a history of GTS was observed to be a risk factor for wheezing among tobacco farmers[13]. However, due to a tolerance effect of nicotine on exposed individuals, the presence of the green tobacco sickness alone is a poor indicator of high levels of nicotine exposure in a population that is chronically exposed to nicotine.

1.2.4.2 Respiratory health effects

Tobacco handling has been associated with different kinds of occupational respiratory problems such as upper and lower respiratory symptoms; compromised lung function indices; including specific conditions like asthma, rhinitis, and COPD[3] as seen in Table 4 below. Most available data are based on factory workers, who work in dusty environments exposed to organic dusts. In addition, exposure to some inorganic dusts in the context of tobacco cultivation predisposes farmers to the health effects associated with inorganic dust exposure which include COPD.

A study among workers in a cigarette factory in Italy observed an association between duration of exposure to tobacco dust and symptoms such as cough, phlegm, wheezing among both smokers and nonsmokers[14].

The study among tobacco processing workers in a Chinese plant revealed a decline in percentage of the predicted pulmonary function compared to controls[15]. Other studies have demonstrated higher percentages (14.3%) of mean diurnal variation in peak expiratory flow among tobacco workers compared to controls (9.8%)[36]. In this study tobacco workers had significantly lower FVC and FEV_1 values compared to controls.

1.2.4.2.1 Asthma and Rhinitis

Pesticides

Studies on pesticide handlers show an increased risk for rhinitis and asthma among this group of workers. Both allergic and non-allergic wheezes have been associated with pesticide application [3,37,38]. Though these studies were not all on tobacco farmers themselves they reveal a potential link that may exist in tobacco farming given the exposure to pesticides in the process of tobacco cultivation.

Tobacco pesticides such as organophosphates, pyrethroids, neonicotinoids, and herbicides have been associated with several respiratory effects. These range from acute symptoms to chronic conditions some of which have been demonstrated in lung function tests. As shown in the table 2 the most common effects are wheezes, rhinitis, as well as atopic and nonatopic asthma[39,40,41,42].

There is consistent evidence that growing up in farms in general is protective for atopic asthma and rhinitis compared to the general population [43–45]. It has further been suggested from those studies that such protection is due to exposure to endotoxins in atopic airway disease.

A review by Ngajilo et al shows the prevalence of rhinitis-like symptoms (nasal congestion, runny nose and itchiness around eyes and nose) among tobacco farmers to be between 8% and 34%[8]. Factors such as harvesting and topping were shown to be associated with runny, stuffy nose in one study. A review [46] focusing on occupational pesticide exposure and respiratory health showed that asthma and chronic bronchitis were associated with pesticide exposure either as an applicator or farmer. Repeated exposure to pesticides was also shown to be associated with increased prevalence of wheeze, which suggests a link between pesticide exposure and airway disease.

Dust role

Studies have shown the role of dust in both upper and lower respiratory symptoms. Ignacak et al. found that chronic or recurrent nasal symptoms were more common among employees exposed to tobacco dust as compared to the control group (40% versus I3.3%, p = 0,018). The exposed population had loss of cilia and squamous epithelial metaplasia compared to controls. However, their tobacco specific IgE did not differ compared to controls and they did not demonstrate hyper-eosinophilia. This suggested that the symptoms were due to irritant effects as opposed to allergic mechanisms.[47] Another Brazilian study evaluating wheezes in tobacco farmers found an association between dust exposure and wheeze[13].

The development of both atopic and irritant induced asthma/rhinitis have been associated with farming [48]. Organic dust exposure from tobacco leaves was associated with wheezing supporting evidence from other studies linking asthma to organic dusts[13]. A case report of a patient with features suggestive of occupational asthma due to dried tobacco leaves exposure has also been reported[8]. In this case, sensitization to tobacco leaf was confirmed by a positive skin-prick test (SPT) using an extract of dried Paraguay Bell leaf. A specific bronchial-challenge test using the same tobacco, not contaminated by mold, was associated with a 23% fall in FEV1. This suggested an IgE dependent sensitisation to tobacco leaf as one of the mechanisms for occupational asthma in tobacco farm workers[8]. Although not many studies have been documented regarding asthma and rhinitis among tobacco workers one can infer a potential for increased risk described in the studies above.

Nicotine role

A Brazilian study on the prevalence of wheezing among tobacco farmers found a greater risk of wheezing associated with lifting sticks with tobacco leaves to be hung in barns, monthly frequency of pesticides use, dry tobacco leaf dust and GTS compared to other tasks of low exposure [13]. From such findings, it can be appreciated that tasks that are likely to increase nicotine exposure are among the risk factors for wheeze in this population.

In the factory setting, a study that assessed both upper and lower airway disease in tobacco factory workers found an increased association between upper airway diseases and dust exposure while the data did not support any association of tobacco dust with lower airway disease [20]. There is need for more quantitative epidemiological evidence of the association with asthma among tobacco farmers since this was the only published study in this setting.

There remains a gap in knowledge on the potential effects of chronic nicotine exposure in agricultural settings on inflammatory response of airways of tobacco farmers.

1.2.4.2.2 COPD and Interstitial lung disease

Pesticides role

An agricultural health study showed that exposure to organophosphates, pyrethroids and other pesticides increased the risk of chronic bronchitis in farmers with Odds Ratios (OR) ranging from 1.41-1.70 depending on the type of pesticides or herbicides used [49]. Although these pesticides do not primarily act on the respiratory system, toxicological studies have revealed adverse health outcomes on the respiratory system related to their use.

Acute exposure effect episodes are very good predictors of occurrence of chronic effects.[50] However, it is not uncommon to observe chronic health effects related to pesticides use among farmers in the absence of preceding acute effects.

Dust role

There is emerging evidence that exposure to silica as well as vapors, gases, dusts, fumes (VGDF) is responsible for a growing global burden of COPD according to research data over the past two decades[51,52,53]. A review by Blanc and others on the relationship of COPD and occupation showed a population attributable fraction of at least 15% of COPD to VGDF. The greater components of these VGDF are classified as low toxicity dusts and, therefore, receive little or no attention in terms of occupational exposure monitoring [54]. The process of tobacco cultivation and processing involves exposure to different forms of VGDF from land preparation to curing, sorting, packaging and selling. Despite this exposure, there is little information on the health effects of VGDF and other associated chemicals on tobacco farmers.

The majority of studies on respiratory diseases of tobacco workers have been conducted in tobacco processing settings where the workers mostly encounter dried tobacco dust. In one study, tobacco plant workers involved in processing tobacco and exposed to dried tobacco dust had an increased risk of developing COPD compared to controls [38]. Similarly, a study conducted in a farm setting using lung function tests of tobacco farm workers exposed to dust, revealed evidence of COPD [55].Tobacco farm workers are exposed to tobacco dust including nicotine and pesticides which could alter the magnitude of COPD burden in that population. In a similar setting a Zimbabwean study among flue-cured tobacco workers showed an increase in COPD cases when compared to vegetable farmers [56].

Nicotine role

In vitro, nicotine has been shown to affect the mucin formation in the airways as well as disrupting the surfactant levels in the lungs [57]. It has been postulated through these mechanisms that nicotine may increase airway resistance and predispose to obstructive pulmonary disease. One study showed that nicotine exposure through tobacco smoke favors proliferation of rat airway smooth muscle cells and could explain its role in obstructive pulmonary disease [58]. Since these studies are mainly laboratory-based trials on animals, it is difficult to determine the exposure levels in the occupational setting that are likely to mimic such effects. Nicotine in tobacco farming is associated with dermal absorption and whilst systemic effects are possible, the mechanism for pulmonary effects are not well understood.

Despite these findings there is limited evidence available for the association of tobacco farming exposures and the prevalence of COPD among tobacco farmers.

Table 1.3: Epidemiological studies of work-related adverse respiratory outcomes in tobacco workers

Study Author and Year	Design and population	Study Aim	Exposure Variables	Outcome Variables	Major Findings
Ngajilo D et al 2018	Literature review	Occupational allergy and asthma in tobacco farmers	Not applicable	Not applicable	Tobacco farming was associated with Rhinitis, asthma, allergic alveolitis, spirometric abnormalities
Fiori N et al 2015	Cross-sectional study of 2469 tobacco farmers In Brazil	Predictors of wheezing in Tobacco Farm workers	Contact with green tobacco, dried tobacco, pesticides, GTS among others	Wheezing	General prevalence of wheezing of 11%. Among men wheezing associated with pesticides use, green tobacco, dried tobacco, strenuous work, age, GTS, smoking. Among women wheezing was associated with contact with tobacco, contact with pesticides, family history of asthma, GTS, strenuous work.
Siavash E et al 2009	Cohort study of 231 exposed and 100 controls In India	Evaluation of Pulmonary function in workers exposed to tobacco dust	Tobacco dust Occupation	Spirometry measurements of lung capacities and air flow	Marked reduction in PEF (78% vs 105%, p<0.001), FEF25% (76% vs 102%, p<0.001), and PIF (75% vs 98%, p<0.001) among the exposed group

Table 1.3: Epidemiological studies of work-related adverse respiratory outcomes in tobacco workers

Study Author and Year	Design and population	Study Aim	Exposure Variables	Outcome Variables	Major Findings
Zhang Y et al 2009	Cross-sectional study 302 exposed and 323 controls In China	Relationship between cumulative dose of tobacco dust exposure and pulmonary injury	Tobacco dust Occupation	Pulmonary function tests (FVC, FEV1, FEF)	Increased abnormalities for both FEV1 and FVC among the exposed group compared to controls (p<0.01 or <0.05)
Chloros D et al 2004	Cross-sectional study 1020 exposed and 469 controls In Greece	Respiratory effects in workers processing dried tobacco leaves	Dried tobacco leaves dust Occupation	Bronchitis Rhinitis COPD	Tobacco workers had a lower prevalence (8.7% vs 20.6%) of bronchitis and higher rhinitis (27.3% vs 17.9%) in workers compared to controls
Jadranka M et al 2003	Cross-sectional n=219 121 exposed and 98 controls In Croatia	Respiratory findings in tobacco workers	Dust Occupation	Asthma symptoms Lung function test Abnormal CXR	6.2% asthma in tobacco workers vs 0 in controls and workers had a lower FEV1 compared to controls

Table 1.3: Epidemiological studies of work-related adverse respiratory outcomes in tobacco workers

Study Author and Year	Design and population	Study Aim	Exposure Variables	Outcome Variables	Major Findings
Flander et al 1988	Cross-sectional study 16 exposed and 32 controls In Denmark	Respiratory disorders among tobacco workers	Tobacco dust occupation	Pulmonary function tests (FVC, FEV1, PEF)	Tobacco workers had significantly lower FVC and FEV1 compared to controls. Tobacco workers had a higher diurnal variation in PEF than controls.
Viegi G et al 1986	Cross-sectional study of 89 men, 93 young women, and 40 older women categorized based on smoking status and work duration Italian farmers	Respiratory effects of occupational exposure to tobacco dust	Tobacco dust Occupation duration (<6years vs >6years) Smoking history (Non-smoker, NS, vs Smokers,S)	Respiratory symptoms such as cough, phlegm, wheeze Pulmonary function tests Chest X-ray findings	Among men, in the order of NS<6, NS>6, S<6, and S>6, chronic cough (4%, 12%, 14%, and 25% respectively; chi square = 4-28, $p < 0.05$), chronic phlegm (9%, 12%, 10%, and 25%; chi square = 4-17, $p < 0.05$), and wheezing (0%, 12%, 29%, and 32%; chi square = 9-84, $p < 0.01$). Pulmonary function tests showed a decreasing but nonsignificant trend with employment duration and smoking
Gosh S et al 1980	Cross-sectional study 290 exposed farmers and 150 control In India	Occupational health problems in agricultural tobacco workers	Tobacco cultivation involving green tobacco, dried tobacco, curing	Green tobacco symptoms Pulmonary function tests (FVC, FEV1) X-ray findings	Significant reduction in FEV1 was noted among the exposed smokers and nonsmokers Greater prevalence of emphysema and TB among exposed subjects

Several factors have been associated with development of respiratory conditions among tobacco farmers. Major factors include host factors such as atopy, gender, comorbidities such as HIV or TB; occupational factors such as job tasks, and environmental factors such as biomass fuel.

1.2.5.1 Host factors

1.2.5.1.1 Atopy

A Norwegian study showed that crop farming is associated with a higher prevalence of atopic asthma compared to animal farming [59]. In a Brazilian study assessing the prevalence of wheezing among tobacco farmers, a family history of asthma was found to be associated with wheezing although existence of atopy was not measured objectively [13]. Generally, there are very few documented studies on atopic factors in crop farm workers, specifically tobacco farmers.

1.2.5.1.2 Sex

A study in Vietnam showed that female farm workers were more likely to have tobacco related symptoms than male counterparts[37]. Although adult onset asthma has been shown to be more common in females, in the Brazilian study of wheezing among tobacco farmers the gender stratified prevalence was the same. It is worth noting, however, that males in this study had more exposures related to asthma risks such as smoking compared to females [13].

1.2.5.1.3 Age

With regard to pesticide use, age was shown to be associated with more severe symptoms among farmers [60]. However, effects of nicotine appear to present with worst symptoms among the population of young farmers [61]. The latter finding, is not consistently demonstrated in many studies as directly related to age per se but rather to years of experience in tobacco cultivation.

1.2.5.1.4 HIV -Status

Although HIV is endemic in most African countries that cultivate tobacco, the burden of HIV among tobacco farmers is not known. It is a well-established fact that HIV increases the risk of developing COPD through exposure to opportunistic infections, altered immune responses and toxic metabolic processes related to anti-retroviral therapy [62–64]. As stated earlier TB which predisposes to the development of COPD is strongly associated with HIV infection. According to WHO, HIV positive individuals are between 26 and 31 times more likely to develop TB infection compared to those without HIV[65-66]. Some studies among HIV infected smokers show that nicotine exposure is associated with increased viral replication, suppressed cell mediated immunity, increased risk of asthma and allergy, and increased risk of COPD [64]. These studies were done on smokers rather than individuals occupationally exposed to nicotine. These studies demonstrated that nicotine was able to do this through its action on nicotinic receptors on immune cells and through the action of its metabolic intermediates on *CYP2A6* [67]. It is not clear whether higher nicotine exposures encountered during tobacco cultivation could have a similar impact on the health of tobacco farmers and whether such an effect may be modified by HIV status.

1.2.5.1.5 Smoking status

Smoking is a major risk factor for asthma and COPD. A study on COPD conducted among adults in urban Malawi revealed a 10.4% prevalence of ever-smoked individuals while other studies have reported a lower population prevalence of 4% [6]. Among Brazilian tobacco farmers the smoking prevalence was dominated by males at 30% compared to females at 3%, and in males this was associated with occurrence of wheeze[13,68,69].

1.2.5.2 Occupational factors

1.2.5.2.1 Job tasks

The Brazilian study on tobacco farmers showed an increased risk of wheezing in men involved with strenuous work and lifting sticks with tobacco leaves to the curing barns[13]. Among the females in that study, strenuous work and tying hands of tobacco were associated with wheezing.

1.2.5.3 Environmental factors

1.2.5.3.1 Biomass Fuel use

Occupational biomass fuel exposure in tobacco cultivation occurs through the fire curing process, bed sterilization when some stubble is burnt on top of the nursery beds.

Tobacco curing carries high risk of exposure to tobacco dust, ammonium, nicotine, carbon monoxide, carbon dioxide, furanic aldehyde, moulds and fungi. The curing process which usually occurs in airtight barns at a constant temperature level (for 72–96 hours), may take up to eight weeks. This requires farmers to constantly enter curing barns to add leaves and branches to an open fire. During this period, farmers inhale large quantities of smoke, which increases their risk of acquiring respiratory disease[8].

There is widespread biomass fuel use (about 90%) in the sub-Saharan African context especially in the rural areas for non-occupational purposes such as everyday cooking [70]. In an urban-based Malawian study, 85.2% of the participants were exposed to biomass fuel through domestic use of firewood, charcoal, or paraffin lamps [6]. Reliance on firewood was associated with significantly higher odds of respiratory and constitutional symptoms such as shortness of breath, difficulty breathing, chest pains, night phlegm, forgetfulness, dizziness, and dry irritated eyes in rural Malawi[71]. Biomass fuel use was associated with ever wheeze in a study done in Nepal[72]. A review by Guoping Hu and others showed an association between biomass fuel use and COPD development in all sexes and Asian as well as non-Asian populations[73]. Since tobacco growing communities are usually remote from the cities, their use of biomass fuel is likely to be higher than the general population.

1.2.6 Conclusion

Available evidence suggests that tobacco famers encounter significant work-related hazardous exposures during the cultivation process, among which are nicotine, pesticides, and particulate dusts. Additionally, tobacco smoke, tuberculosis, and biomass fuel exposure are being increasingly recognized as important risk factors for chronic lung disease in developing countries[74]. While all these exposures have been linked to the development of chronic respiratory disease, the effect of concomitant exposures to these agents in a setting of high HIV prevalence needs to be evaluated. Knowledge generated from such a study is needed to inform intervention programs aimed at controlling all these factors to minimize the occurrence of chronic respiratory disease among tobacco farmers.

CHAPTER 2: AIMS, OBJECTIVE AND METHODS

2.1 JUSTIFICATION AND PURPOSE

Although a body of literature exists that deals with acute health effects of nicotine and pesticides among tobacco farmers, there remains a huge gap in knowledge about their chronic effects. Moreover, very few studies have attempted to study the associations of such exposures with respiratory disease occurrence. Among those that have studied respiratory health effects, most have lacked objective measurement tools in their assessment of exposures and outcomes. This study focusses on the association between respiratory health and tobacco farming among Malawian farmers with concomitant exposure to nicotine in tobacco leaves and pesticides.

This study adopts a more objective approach to quantifying the prevalence of COPD and asthma among tobacco farmers and determining the role of nicotine and pesticide exposure in the occurrence of these conditions. This will be carried out in the context of identifying and controlling for potential confounders implicated in the development of these conditions. In this particular setting, factors to be considered are the roles of HIV status, biomass fuel use, smoking, and previous tuberculosis episode. Although the majority of farmers cultivate burley tobacco, there are several occupational health and social protection implications associated with flue cured tobacco by the nature of the employment in such large estates as well as the magnitude of workplace exposures associated with their specific working conditions.

This is the first study, to our knowledge, that attempts to evaluate the effect of concurrent exposure to nicotine and pesticides on the prevalence of respiratory disease in the context of a HIV prevalence among flue cured tobacco farmers in Malawi.

The findings of this study would help to inform recommendations on the control of risk factors associated with development of obstructive lung disease among tobacco farmers in the Malawian setting and similar contexts in Sub-Saharan Africa.

2.2 HYPOTHESIS

Concurrent exposure to nicotine and pesticides during tobacco cultivation increases the risk of developing obstructive lung disease among flue cured tobacco farmers.

2.3 RESEARCH QUESTIONS

1. What are the respiratory health effects of individuals with concurrent exposure to nicotine and pesticides among tobacco farmers in Malawi?
2. What is the prevalence of obstructive lung disease and lung function impairment in Malawian tobacco farmers?
3. How does HIV infection, biomass fuel combustion exposures, pulmonary tuberculosis (PTB), and smoking contribute to the prevalence of obstructive lung disease among tobacco farmers?

2.4 AIM

To determine the association between concurrent exposure to nicotine and pesticides with measures of obstructive lung disease among flue cured tobacco farmers in Zomba district of Malawi.

2.5 OBJECTIVES

1. To determine the prevalence of obstructive lung disease (asthma and COPD) among a population of tobacco farmers in Malawi
2. To describe the exposure to nicotine and pesticides in this population using self-reported indices of exposure
3. To evaluate the role of nicotine and pesticide exposure as well as additional factors associated with potentially increased risk for obstructive lung disease in this population such as gender, smoking status, HIV status, previous tuberculosis episode, exposure to biomass fuel.

2.6 METHODS

2.6.1 Study design

This was a cross sectional study targeting all the estate farmer worker population of >18 years of age working on four estate farms in Malawi between December, 2017 and January 2018. This study was conducted during spraying and topping season which also includes some weeding.

2.6.2 Study population

Zomba district is located in the southern part of Malawi where there are at least 15 large flue cured tobacco estates[75] and some small holder farmers which, together constituted a population of 5000 tobacco workers. The workers studied in this district were estate employees of four large tobacco estates. Flue cured tobacco farmers were considered an appropriate population that would allow measurement of all the exposures considered in this study due to the very nature of the cultivation process. Zomba provided a convenient source of flue cured tobacco estates.

2.6.3 Sampling strategy

Participants were selected from the largest estates of the district based on the Tobacco Control Commission employment statistics. The four neighbouring largest estates that include flue curing as part of the tobacco process were chosen. These employ between 80 (on the smallest farm) and 350 (on the largest farm) seasonal workers each year. All available farm workers during a shift aged 18 years and above within these tobacco estates were invited to participate. Invitations were made to all departments in order to have representation from all departments.

2.6.4 Sample size

A Brazilian study among tobacco farmers reported a prevalence of 3 to 28% for asthma-like symptoms[138]. Other local studies in Malawi on a non-farming community reported a 10% prevalence for an obstructive lung function. The sample size therefore assumed a prevalence of obstructive lung disease (COPD and asthma) in this population to be 10%[76]. Further consideration for computing sample size is the population size of about 5,000 in the Zomba district and using a 95% confidence level. Using an online sample size calculator[77,78] the sample size needed for determining the population prevalence was 357 participants .

Health outcome assessment

Questionnaire

Each participant answered a modified European Community Respiratory Health Survey II questionnaire (Appendix 1). The questionnaire was modified for local conditions and was also translated into Chichewa and back translated to assess validity and reproducibility. The questionnaire was administered by trained interviewers. The questionnaire was designed to be completed within 30-40 minutes and had various components. The questionnaire included participant's demographic characteristics such as age, gender, seniority, smoking habits and occupational information. Standardized questions were asked about respiratory symptoms and history of respiratory disease. This included asthma and COPD- related symptoms such as wheeze, tight chest, cough and shortness of breath and rhino conjunctivitis symptoms such as sneezing, itchy eyes and blocked nose. The questionnaire was supplemented with questions relating to the history of a participant's asthma (medication used, asthma attacks, doctor visits). Occupational information focused on the job history, workplace setting, job tasks and duration and frequency of exposure to nicotine and pesticide. Questions on other potential risk factors for the development of obstructive lung disease such as: family history of atopy; smoking history, use of biomass fuel, and previous TB episode were included.

Spirometry

All interviewed workers were subjected to spirometry at the end of their shifts and all American Thoracic Society (ATS)/ERS guidelines for conducting spirometry were followed[79]. The EasyOn PC Spirometer was used. It utilizes digital ultrasonic flow measurement technology, which ensures accurate results, repeatable performance and quality control. Trained nurses conducted spirometry of 10 individuals on average per day. Spirometry was performed in a sitting position without a nose clip. Each worker performed up to eight trials to produce three acceptable curves. Test reproducibility was used as a guide to whether further attempts will be necessary. Reproducibility criteria was the two best tracings for both FEV1 and FVC varying by no more than 150 ml or 5%, whichever was greater. However, failure to meet reproducibility criteria did not result in exclusion of the spirogram results from the statistical analysis. Poor reproducibility may also be an independent marker of airway dysfunction. Technologist/testers were trained to ensure the quality of spirograms.

The lung function indices of primary interest included forced vital capacity (FVC) and forced expiratory volume in one second (FEV1). The best FEV1 and FVC were used regardless of whether they belonged to the same tracing. Lung volumes obtained by spirometry were adjusted for body temperature and pressure according to the temperature and atmospheric pressure measured on a continuous basis throughout the day. Reference values of the National Health and Nutrition Examination Survey III were used for spirometry interpretation, with lower limits corresponding to the 95th percentile. Heights and weights of workers were recorded for calculating predicted lung function indices using National health and Nutrition Examination Survey III (NHANES III) equations. Workers were provided with special instructions to ensure that tested individuals do not smoke tobacco (at least 2 hours before) and do not take any anti-asthmatic inhalers (12 hours before) or oral asthma medications (48 hours before) prior to the test. The results of lung function tests were recorded on a lung function tests data collection sheet (Appendix 6).

iii) HIV Status

HIV status was determined by first self-reporting and verification by requesting consent to check the health passport documentation. Where the participant has not had any previous provider- initiated test, such counselling and testing was offered using HIV rapid test kits with outcomes stated as positive or negative or unknown (categorical variable). Participants who tested positive were appropriately referred for further care and counselling.

Exposure assessment:

Qualitative health risk assessment per farm

A brief walk-through survey with the estate supervisor/manager was done to evaluate and familiarize the researcher with the occupational setting. Aspects that were assessed included : farm size, prevalent hazards related to tobacco cultivation and work practices: number of employees, hours of work, list of chemicals used, seasonality of exposure, etc on each farm. Questions related to tobacco handling practices (sowing, transplanting, pest control, harvesting, curing and stacking) were included to arrive at a qualitative understanding of exposure and different phases involved in tobacco farming.

2.6.6 Data management and analysis

Questionnaire data was collected electronically using digital tablets. All data collected through questionnaires and testing results were compiled and entered into STATA 14. Questionnaires were coded for double entry by the Information Technology Services at the Johns Hopkins Project. Each individual who agreed to participate was assigned a unique code. The database with data input from the questionnaires was analyzed using STATA version 14. Independent checks of range, validity, consistency and missing data was performed. Logic check programs were run to ensure that each value found in the data fell within the expected range or correspond to possible values in the codebook and the study coordinator resolved discrepancies.

Key associations of interest involved investigating relationships between the occupational risk factor and the health outcomes. The key variables of interest are listed below.

2.6.6.1 Dependent variables

1. Symptom based definitions based on respiratory questionnaire were used in determining respiratory health outcomes:

   - Symptom based diagnosis of chronic bronchitis (COPD): Cough and sputum on most days lasting at least 3 months for two consecutive years
   - ECRHS Asthma definition: defined as either having shortness of breath in the past 12 months or an asthma attack in the past 12 months or current use of asthma medication
   - Asthma symptom score: An asthma symptom score was computed based on the sum of answers (0=no, 1=yes) to five questions on asthma-like symptoms in the past 12 months (short of breath while wheezing, woken up with chest tightness, attack of shortness of breath at rest, attack of shortness of breath after exercise, woken up by attack of shortness of breath). Asthma was positive if yes to ≥ 2 questions.

- In addition Work-related chest symptoms and work-related nasal-ocular symptoms were also treated as outcomes of interest

2. Results of lung function results were also used to define airway obstruction in respiratory health outcomes:

   A. FEV1<Lower Limit of Normal (LLN): Based on the Global Lung Initiative (GLI) equation
   B. FEV1<80%: this was based on the comparison with NHANES III reference values
   C. FEV1/FVC<LLN: Based on the Global Lung Initiative (GLI) equation

   D. FEV1/FVC <70%: this was determined by using a standard cut-off of 70% for ratio
   E. Moderate to severe obstruction: defined as FEV1<80% and FEV1/FVC<70%

2.6.6.2 Independent variables

Nicotine exposure

The main exposure variables for nicotine exposure were GTS symptoms, tasks involving contact with tobacco e.g. weeding, topping, harvesting, hanging tobacco, sorting, grading, stacking and related tasks.

Pesticide exposure history

These variables include working with pesticides, cleaning spraying equipment, working near pesticide applicators, getting into the field soon after spraying, pesticide drift into the home, use of tobacco pesticides at home, and related tasks.

2.6.6.3 Confounding factors and covariates:

Potential occupational covariates that were considered were host factors such as: age, gender, smoking status, family history of asthma, use of biomass fuel, HIV status and previous TB episode.

2.6.7 Statistical analysis

STATA statistical package version 14 was utilized for data management and calculating descriptive, bivariate, univariate and multivariate regression statistics, where appropriate. Exploratory data analysis was carried out to highlight general features of the data that would guide further analysis. This included running descriptive checks that would reveal the number of observations, the type of variables, presence of outliers, the nature of data cleaning required and the extent of missing data as well as the distributions of the key variables. The data was then cleaned as required, missing variables labeled accordingly and outliers censored. Descriptive statistics were used to stratify the occupational groups and to analyze the independent variables amongst those groups. Univariate analyses were used to summarize the distribution of each measured variable. Exploratory bivariate analyses were used to assess the nature of the associations between exposures, outcomes and covariates. Multivariate regression analysis was applied to examine the association between the dependent and independent variables. Confounding and effect modification by covariates were considered in the formulation of the models.

2.7 ETHICS

The researcher sought approval from both the University of Cape Town Health Sciences Faculty Research Ethics Committee (HREC) as well as the Research Ethics Committee of the College of Medicine in Malawi (COMREC) and was carried out based on the following ethical principles:

2.7.1 Autonomy

An informed consent was sought after which individuals were free to participate or not at no associated cost. Appendix1.

2.7.2 Confidentiality

The research data for participants was treated with utmost confidentiality and communication of their test results were made directly to them. No personal identifiers were used and the information was not accessed by individuals who were not part of the investigating team.

2.7.3 Benefit

At individual level the participants were aware of their health outcomes and those with concerns were referred to their doctors. Furthermore, the findings of this research would help to inform appropriate measures for minimizing the burden of obstructive lung disease among tobacco farmers.

2.7.4 No harm

We anticipated a negligible risk to arise during the course of the research to the participants except for discomfort coming from sample collections, spirometry, but they were allowed to withdraw where they experienced too much discomfort. Participants with abnormal findings were communicated with and counselled regarding their condition and where necessary the employer was advised with regard to workplace accommodation (with consent from the participant).

2.7.5 Justice

The growing concern of tobacco farmers' exposure to pesticides and nicotine and scanty information about the effects on them justified carrying out this particular research in this population. It was anticipated that this would provide us with specific information that will inform recommended interventions needed to improve their working conditions to minimize health risk.

2.8 RESEARCH FINDINGS AND DISSEMINATION OF RESULTS

The findings from the study quantify the prevalence and burden of obstructive lung disease among tobacco farmers. It identifies and characterizes significant associations related to tobacco and pesticide exposure and other risk factors and will help to make informed decisions aimed at preventing and controlling obstructive lung diseases and their risk factors in this population.

- It forms the basis of an MPhil book
- Conference presentations will be made
- Publication in scientific journal
- Report to the Tobacco Commission and Funder

CHAPTER 3: RESULTS

3.1 Population and demographic characteristics

A total of four farms were contacted with a total number of 759 seasonal perennial workers. Due to variations in farm activities during the calendar only about 60% of the population were called for duties during the study period which occurred during the spraying and topping season. All available employees were briefed about the survey and were to take part at the end of their shift by reporting to the administration offices where interviews and tests were conducted. A total of 281 employees consented to participate. Of these, 279 completed the questionnaire while 276 attempted spirometry. Among those who consented for spirometry 258 performed spirometry successfully while 18 did not complete. No participant had satisfied any exclusion criteria for spirometry among those who were interviewed.

Table 3.1a: Study participation rate

	Farm 1	Farm 2	Farm 3	Farm 4
Total number of employees n=759 (%)	350(46)	162(21)	167(22)	80(11)
Consented to participate n=281 (% of particular farm population)	183(52)	25(15)	35(21)	38(48)
Interviewed n=279 (% of particular farm population)	183(52)	23(14)	35(21)	38(48)
Completed spirometry n=258 (% of particular farm population)	173(49)	21(13)	31(19)	33(41)

As seen from the table 3.1a above farm 1 and 4 had better participation rate than farms 2 and 3. The main reasons were farm logistics and employee engagement with supervisory staff. We observed that farms 1 and 4 had a good relation between supervisory staff and employees and it was easier to mobilize and address the employees than was the case with the other two farms.

Data from the 279 farmers from all the four farms was analyzed. As shown in table 3.1b below, the average age was 37.7±12.6 years and the majority were males (68%). Most of the participants (73%) had attained at least a primary education but there was a significant association between education and gender (p=0.000) with greater proportion of males attending more years of education than females.

The majority of respondents were non-smokers (73%) with 20% current smokers while 7% had quit smoking. Cannabis use was prevalent among 5% of the farmers in this population. Alcohol use was reported by 42%.

Among the participants, 16% of them were tested positive or reported a previous positive test for HIV. Some participants did not know their HIV status because they declined an offer to be tested and had not been tested before (18%).

With respect to previous respiratory illness, 10% of the participants reported a history of repeated childhood chest infections, 4% reported a t history of previous pulmonary tuberculosis while 3% had suffered chronic bronchitis before.

Table 3.1b: Demographic characteristics of tobacco farmers in Malawi

Demographic characteristic	Baseline Prevalence (%) n =279	Male n=189 (68)	Female n=90 (32)	p-value
*Age (years)	37.7±12.6	37.8 (35.9-39.7)	37.4 (35.1-39.6)	0.787
Home Language				0.637
- Lhomwe	123(44)	87 (46)	36 (40)	
- Yao	40(14)	28 (14)	12 (13)	
- Sena	1(0.3)	1 (1)	0	
- Chichewa	0(0)	0	0	
- Other	115(41)	73 (39)	42 (47)	
Education				**0.000**
- None	30(11)	9 (4.8)	21 (23.3)	
- Lower primary	86(31)	49 (25.9)	37 (41.1)	
- Upper primary	117(42)	87 (46.0)	30 (33.3)	
- Secondary	46(16)	44 (23.3)	2 (2.2)	
Smoking status: n (%)				
- Current smokers	57(20)	39 (20.6)	18(20.0)	0.902
- Ex-smokers	19(7)	15(8)	4(4)	0.279
- Never smokers	203(73)	135(71)	68(76)	0.469
Cannabis use	14(5)	10(5)	4(4)	0.762
Alcohol	118(42)	82(43)	36(40)	0.593
- Ever felt need to reduce alcohol	84(30)	55(29)	29(32)	0.595
- Ever felt guilty due to drinking	72(26)	49(26)	23(26)	0.947
- Ever criticized of drinking	56(20)	38(20)	18(20)	0.984
- Having to get early morning drinks	44(16)	29(15)	15(17)	0.777
HIV status				0.115
- Negative (reported or tested)	184(66)	132 (69.4)	52 (57.8)	
- Positive (reported or tested)	44(16)	25 (13.2)	19 (21.1)	
- Unknown	51(18)	32 (16.9)	19 (21.1)	
Past medical history				
- Repeated childhood chest infections	29(10)	23(12)	6(7)	0.159
- Previous TB episode	10(4)	7(4)	3(3)	1.000
- Chronic bronchitis	9(3)	7(4)	2(2)	0.723

*Presented as mean and standard deviation

3.2 Farm and occupational characteristics

Participants were drawn from, four tobacco farms with an annual production ranging from 80 to 250 tones (Table 3.2a). The main type of tobacco cultivated was the flue cured variety which was handled by 99 percent of the participants. The other reported varieties were Burley and Northern Division Dark Fire-Cured (NDDF). Two thirds of respondents came from the largest farm among the four due to logistical issues and accessibility of the farmers.

Table 3.2a: General farm descriptions

Farm name	Farm size	Tobacco quantity	Total number of employees	Total study employees	Male employees	Female employees
Farm 1	210	250	350	183(66)	124(66)	59(66)
Farm 2	132	150	162	23(8)	20(11)	3(3)
Farm 3	90	110	167	35(13)	27(14)	8(9)
Farm 4	74	80	80	38(14)	18(10)	20(22)

The median duration of employment for the farmers was 5 years with a significantly lower duration of 4 years among females than males (5 years). Among the respondents 62% reported working mainly with tobacco, 20% of the workers worked mainly with pesticides in their job, 4% were supervisors while the rest did some construction related work such as wielding, building and plumbing. About 28% of the workers indicated to handle both tobacco and pesticides in their job tasks regardless of their job description. Only 22% of the farmers reported use of protective equipment at work while 20% indicated that their protective equipment is provided by the employer for free. The main task for which protective equipment was worn was spraying of chemicals as reported by 15% of the respondents. Masks, aprons, gloves and goggles were the commonly used protective equipment (Table 3.2b). There were no significant associations in the tasks and use of PPE with gender.

Table 3.2b: Workplace characteristics

Farm and Occupational characteristics	Baseline Prevalence (%) n =279	Baseline Prevalence (%) n =189 Males	Baseline Prevalence (%) n =90 Females	p-value
Types of tobacco cultivated				
Flue cured	276(99)			
Burley- air-cured	5(2)			
Northern division dark fire-cured (NDDF)	1(0.0)			
Types of job				0.671
- Tobacco handler	174(62)	118(63)	56(62)	
- Chemical handler	56(20)	40(21)	16(18)	
- Supervisor	10(4)	5(3)	5(5)	
- Other (plumbing, building, cooking, welder)	37(13)	24(13)	13(15)	
Work with tobacco & pesticides	77(28)	56(30)	21(23)	0.271
Employment duration*	5 (2-10)	5 (2-10)	4 (2-8)	**0.031**
Availability of washrooms at workplace	172(62)	113(60)	59(68)	0.239
Availability of handwashing facilities at workplace	40(14)	23(12)	17(20)	0.114
Personal Protective Equipment (PPE) use	61(22)	44(23)	17(19)	0.407
Tasks during which PPE is used				
- Spraying	43(15)	32(17)	11(12)	0.538
- Curing	12(4)	9(5)	3(3)	1.000
- Sorting	5(2)	2(1)	3(3)	0.181
- Tilling	4(1)	3(2)	1(1)	1.000
- Harvesting	3(1)	2(1)	1(1)	1.000
- Sowing, Transplant, weeding	2(1)	2(1)	0	0.327
- Stacking	2(1)	1(1)	1(1)	0.483
- Cleaning equipment (including PPE)	2(1)	2(1)	0	0.489
- Other tasks including transport, administration	14(5)	10(5)	4(4)	0.876
PPE regularly for at least a year				
- Mask	44(16)	31(16)	13(14)	0.675
- Gloves	37(13)	26(14)	11(12)	0.724
- Apron	20(7)	14(7)	6(7)	0.823
- Goggles	20(7)	13(7)	7(8)	0.785
- Others (boots)	9(3)	8(4)	1(1)	0.168
Free provision of PPE by employer	56(20)	40(21)	16(18)	0.509

*Presented as median and interquartile range

3.3 Respiratory symptoms

As shown in table 3.3 the prevalence of those who reported to ever have asthma was 8% with the majority having their asthma before age of 17 (88%). There was a significant association between childhood asthma and gender with more males reporting childhood asthma than females. Using an ECRHS definition 20% of respondents met the criteria for possible current asthma whilst 23% had an asthma score of ≥2 in keeping with a diagnosis of possible asthma. The prevalence of asthma related symptoms in the past 12 months ranged from 8% to 30% with the most common symptoms being reported as shortness of breath following exercise (30%); attacks of wheezing (19%); shortness of breath and wheezing (19%) and shortness of breath during daytime (18%).

The prevalence of childhood hay fever was 6%. Nasal-ocular symptoms were reported by 29% of the respondents. Additionally, eye symptoms were shown to significantly affect more females than males, 28% and 16%, respectively.

COPD prevalence was 17% based on a standard definition although 10-33% of respondents reported a history of COPD symptoms.

Table 3.3: Self-reported respiratory and nasal-ocular symptoms by tobacco farmers in Malawi

Symptom	Baseline Prevalence (%) n=279	Baseline Prevalence Male (%) n=189	Baseline Prevalence Female (%) n=90	p-value
Asthma history				
Ever had asthma (self-reported known)	23(8)	19(10)	4(4)	0.111
Asthma at ≤ 16 years	19(7)	17(9)	2(2)	**0.036**
Asthma > 16 years	3(1)	1(1)	2(2)	0.200
Current Asthma (ECRHS definition)	55(20)	40(21)	15	0.377
Woken up by an attack of shortness of breath in the last 12 months	50(18)	35(19)	15(17)	0.706
Asthma attack in the past 12 months	9(3)	8(4)	1(1)	0.168
Current use of asthma medication	3(1)	2(1)	1(1)	0.968
Doctor-diagnosed asthma	4(1)	3(2)	1(1)	0.754
Childhood hay fever	16(6)	12(6)	4(4)	0.522
Childhood asthma	19(7)	17(9)	2(2)	**0.036**
Asthma-related symptoms				
Ever had attacks of wheezing (wheezing in the past)	68(24)	47(25)	21(23)	0.780
Wheezing in the past 12 months	54(19)	38(20)	16(18)	0.645
Shortness of breath while wheezing in the last 12 months	54(19)	38(20)	16(18)	0.645
Wheezing or whistling without cold / flu symptoms	40(14)	29(15)	11(12)	0.487
Woken up with chest tightness in the last 12 months	23(8)	16(8)	7(8)	0.845
Attack of shortness of breath at rest during daytime in the last 12 months	50(18)	35(19)	15(17)	0.706
Attack of shortness of breath following running or exercise in the last 12 months	83(30)	54(29)	29(32)	0.533
Asthma symptom score*				0.754
Asthma Score of 0-1	214(77)	146(77)	68(76)	
Asthma Score of 2-5	65(23)	43(23)	22(24)	
Upper airway symptoms				
Presence of nasal-ocular symptoms ever	82(29)	50(26)	32(36)	0.119
≥2 episodes in past 12 months				
- Nasal	36(13)	21(11)	15(17)	0.196
- Eyes	56(20)	31(16)	25(28)	**0.027**
COPD symptoms History				
Woken up by attack of cough or phlegm in last 12 months	91(33)	60(32)	31(34)	0.653
Usual cough first thing in morning	61(22)	39(21)	22(24)	0.472
Day / night cough	55(20)	35(19)	20(22)	0.467
Cough on most days / nights for 3 or more months a year in each of last 2 years	36(13)	22(12)	14(16)	0.362
Phlegm on most days / nights for 3 or more months a year in each of last 2 years	28(10)	17(9)	11(12)	0.402
Chronic bronchitis: Cough or phlegm on most days / nights for 3 or more months a year in each of last 2 years	48(17)	29(15)	19(21)	0.233
Phlegm first thing in morning	52(19)	32(17)	20(22)	0.289
Day/ night phlegm	46(16)	26(14)	20(22)	0.075
Trouble with breathing	52(19)	36(19)	16(18)	0.799
- rarely	33(12)	23(12)	10(11)	
- repeatedly	14(5)	10(5)	4(4)	
- continuously	5(2)	3(2)	2(2)	

*Asthma symptom score: An asthma symptom score was computed based on the sum of answers (0=no, 1=yes) to five questions on asthma-like symptoms in the past 12 months (short of breath while wheezing, woken up with chest tightness, attack of shortness of breath (SOB) at rest, attack of shortness of breath after exercise, woken up by attack of shortness of breath)

#Current asthma attack of SOB in the last 12 months or asthma attack in the last 12 months or current use of asthma medication (ECRHS definition)

3.4 Work-related respiratory symptoms

The respondents demonstrated a higher prevalence of work- related chest symptoms (29%) with 11% reporting an episode of high exposure at work as causing respiratory symptoms. Reported causes of the work related chest symptoms were exposure to dried tobacco (12%), smoke from fires (5%), soil dust (5%), pesticides (4%) and farming in the field (4%). A few (4%) of the respondents reported switching jobs due to chest symptoms.

Work related nasal-ocular symptoms were less common (20%) and were caused by exposure to pesticides (8%), soil dust (5%) and dried tobacco (4%). Table 3.4. No associations were observed between work-related respiratory symptoms and gender.

Table 3.4: Work-related symptoms reported by tobacco farmers in Malawi

Symptom	Baseline Prevalence (%) n = 279	Baseline Prevalence (%) n=189	Baseline Prevalence (%) n=90	p-value
Work-related chest symptoms				
Episode of high exposure at work causing tight chest, shortness of breath, wheeze or cough	30(11)	19(10)	11(12)	0.585
Work-related chest symptoms (ever) [a]	80(29)	58(31)	22(24)	0.281
Job change due to work-related chest symptoms	10(4)	9 (5)	1(1)	0.125
Common causes of chest symptoms				0.337
- Dried tobacco	33(12)	21(11)	12(13)	
- Dust (soil)	15(5)	10(5)	5(6)	
- Smoke from fire	13(5)	10(5)	3(3)	
- Pesticides	12(4)	11(6)	1(1)	
- Farming in the field	10(4)	9(5)	1(1)	
Work-related upper airway symptoms				
Work-related nasal-ocular symptoms	57(20)	33(17)	24(27)	0.075
Causes of nasal-ocular symptoms				0.814
- Pesticides	22(8)	14(7)	8(9)	
- Dust (soil)	14(5)	9(5)	5(6)	
- Dried tobacco	11(4)	6(3)	5(6)	
- Fresh tobacco	3(1)	2(1)	1(1)	
- Farming in the field	2(1)	1(1)	1(1)	

[a] Symptoms chest experienced at work ever

3.5 Exposure to biomass fuel

Table 3.5 demonstrates the environmental and occupational exposure to biomass fuel. Most of the farmers (87%) had daily exposure to biomass fuel for an average of 3 hours. The prevalence of work- related exposure only was 17% while 42% are exposed to biomass fuel at home only, with27% of the farmers reporting a combined exposure to biomass at home and work. The main fuel used was firewood and the two main tasks associated with biomass fuel exposure were cooking (78%) and curing of tobacco (44%). There was no observed significant association between exposure to biomass fuels and gender.

Table 3.5: Biomass fuel exposure of tobacco farmers in Malawi

Environmental and occupational exposure	Baseline Prevalence (%) n = 279	Baseline Prevalence (%) n=189	Baseline Prevalence (%) n=90	p-value
Biomass fuel				
Exposed to biomass fuels	242 (87)	166(88)	76(84)	0.436
- Home only	118(42)	85(45)	33(37)	0.218
- Work only	48 (17)	34(18)	14(16)	0.615
- Both home and work	76(27)	47(25)	29(32)	0.197
Main source				0.499
- Firewood	241(86)	165(87)	76(84)	
- Charcoal	1 (0)	1(1)	0	
- Coal	0(0)	0	0	
- Other	0(0)	0	0	
Main tasks exposing to environmental smoke at home/work or both				
- Cooking	218(78)	147(78)	71(79)	0.834
- Curing (flue)	123(44)	79(42)	44(49)	0.305
- Smoke from tobacco	13(5)	8(4)	5(6)	0.476
- Other	1(0.0)	1(1)	0	0.489
Frequency of exposure to biomass*				
- Hours per day(IQR)	3(2-6)	3(2-6)	3(2-6)	0.478
- Days per month(IQR)	30(30-30)	30 (30-30)	30(30-30)	0.067
- Months per year(IQR)	12(12-12)	12(12-12)	12(12-12)	0.638
- Days per year (IQR)	365(360-365)	365(360-365)	365(365-365)	0.171

*Presented as median and interquartile range

3.6 Nicotine exposure

The presence of green tobacco sickness (GTS) was used as a proxy for acute nicotine exposure and toxicity. The prevalence of GTS in the previous year was 26% and participants reported an average of 3 episodes occurring in that period. The majority of symptoms (24%) occurred on the same day of exposure. Headache and nausea were the commonly reported symptoms, 29% and 17% respectively. Nausea and vomiting were significantly higher among males than females while the rest of the symptoms did not show any association with gender. Harvesting, curing, and sowing were the key tasks that were linked to GTS symptoms.

Table 3.6: Nicotine exposure of tobacco farmers in Malawi

Environmental and occupational exposure	Baseline Prevalence (%) n = 279	Baseline Prevalence (%) n=189	Baseline Prevalence (%) n=90	p-value
Nicotine exposure				
GTS symptoms ever	98(35)	69(37)	29(32)	0.483
GTS Symptoms in past 12 months	73(26)	53(28)	20(22)	0.301
GTS Symptoms				
- Headache	81(29)	53(28)	28(31)	0.598
- Nausea	47(17)	38(20)	9(10)	**0.035**
- Dizziness	29(10)	21(11)	8(9)	0.570
- Vomiting	16(6)	15(8)	1(1)	**0.022**
How many episodes of GTS in the last 12 months‡	3.2±1	3.1(2)	3.5	0.181
How soon after work did symptoms occur				0.582
- Same day	67(24)	49(26)	18(20)	
- Day after	6(2)	3(2)	3(3)	
- 2 days after	7(3)	6(3)	1(1)	
- 3 days after	4(1)	3(2)	1(1)	
- A week after	14(5)	8(4)	6(7)	
Farm activities associated with GTS symptoms				
- Harvesting	50(18)	32(17)	18(20)	0.532
- Curing	31(11)	18(10)	13(14)	0.221
- Sowing	28(10)	21(11)	7(8)	0.386
- Transplanting	23(8)	15(8)	8(9)	0.787
- Other (uprooting, planting, grading)	30(11)	25(13)	5(6)	0.053

‡ presented as mean and standard deviation

3.7   Pesticides exposure

Table 3.7 outlines the participants' exposure characteristics to pesticides. More than half (57%) of the farmers reported application of pesticides in their job for approximately 1 hour per day for 60 days a year. Many of the farmers (72%) reported pesticide exposure during spraying and 83% re-entered the fields soon after spraying pesticides. The commonest pesticides used were organophosphates (18%) followed by copper (15%), and pyrethroids (8%). About half of the farmers report the use of pesticides at their homes including tobacco pesticides (15%) and other domestic pesticides (39%). Farmers also indicated that they use organophosphate pesticides to preserve their grains at home (37%).

Table 3.7: Pesticides exposure of tobacco farmers in Malawi

Environmental and occupational exposure	Baseline Prevalence (%) n = 279	Baseline Prevalence (%) n=189	Baseline Prevalence (%) n=90	p-value
Pesticide exposure				
Pesticides application	158(57)	111(59)	47(52)	0.305
Work near pesticides sprayers	200 (72)	135(71)	65(72)	0.891
- #Number of days worked in the field near sprayers while pesticides are applied per season	14.0±22	13.8±19	14.5±27	0.820
*Frequency of pesticide use among				
- Hours per day(IQR)	1(1-1)	1(1-1)	1(1-1)	0.885
- Days per month(IQR)	24(12-30)	24(8-30)	24(12-30)	0.996
- Days per year use pesticides(IQR)	60(30-120)	60(30-150)	60(30-100)	0.403
Pesticide types				
- Organophosphates	49(18)	36(19)	13(14)	0.345
- Copper	42(15)	30(16)	12(13)	0.406
- Pyrethroids	23(8)	18(10)	5(6)	0.260
- Neonicotinoids	4(1)	3(2)	1(1)	0.754
- Herbicides	3(1)	3(2)	0	0.229
- Other (decanol, benomyl, pyraclostrobin, fluopyram)	48(32)	34(18)	14(16)	0.406
Exposure during spraying	45 (16)	26(14)	19(21)	0.118
Pesticide drift	22 (8)	12(6)	10(11)	0.168
Field re-entry soon after spraying	232 (83)	158(84)	74(82)	0.774
Home use of pesticides	142 (51)	94(50)	48(53)	0.574
Types of pesticides used at home				
o Tobacco pesticides used at home	42(15)	27(14)	15(17)	0.603
- Actellic (organophosphorus-pirimiphos methyl)	104(37)	68(36)	36(40)	0.760
- Pesticides for tomato plants (not specified)	1(0.0)	1(1)	0	
- Maize pills	1(0.0)	1(1)	0	
- Servin (carbamate)	1(0.0)	1(1)	0	
- Unknown (used for ticks)	1(0.0)	1(1)	0	

* *Presented as median and interquartile range
#Presented as mean and standard deviation

3.8 Pulmonary function tests

Spirometry results were available for 258 participants and were interpreted using NHANES and Global Lung Initiative (GLI) criteria. The median FEV_1 was 2.64L(2.15L-3.13L) and showed a significant association with gender with female indices lower compared to males. Using NHANES references, 20% of the participants had an FEV1 below 80% of the predicted value suggesting an element of airflow limitation. When GLI equations were used to determine those with FEV_1<LLN the prevalence was 31% and showed significant association with gender with a higher proportion of females affected. The median ratio (FEV1/FVC) was 80.89 (IQR: 76.03-85.23) which was within the normal range with 8% of the respondents having a ratio of less than 70% suggestive of airway obstruction.

Using GLI criteria, 31% had an FEV1 < LLN and 28% had an FVC<LLN, with 14% having an FEV1/FVC<LLN in keeping with possible airflow limitation. The median percentage of predicted values for FEV1 and FVC were higher when using NHANES than when using GLI, 95% and 96% versus 86% and 89%, respectively.

Table 3.8: Pulmonary function indices of Tobacco farmers in Malawi

Pulmonary function indices*	Prevalence (%) n=258	Male Baseline Prevalence (%) n=179	Female Baseline Prevalence (%) n=79	p-value	Prevalence (%) n=258	Male Baseline Prevalence (%) n=179	Female Baseline Prevalence (%) n=79	p-value
	BASELINE NHANES				BASELINE GLI			
FEV$_1$ L [median (IQR)]	2.64 (2.15 – 3.13)	2.93 (2.43-3.32)	2.1 (1.83-2.40)	**0.000**	2.64 (2.15 – 3.13)	2.93 (2.43-3.32	2.1 (1.83-2.40)	**0.000**
FVC L [median (IQR)]	3.29 (2.67-3.86)	3.59 (3.12-3.99)	2.62 (2.37-2.92)	**0.000**	3.29 (2.67-3.86)	3.59 (3.12-3.99)	2.62 (2.37-2.92)	**0.000**
FEV$_1$ % pred. [median (IQR)]	95.46 (82.38-105.00)	98.03 (83.63-105.17)	89.57 (81.45-104.74)	0.329	85.66(74.89-94.61)	87.11 (75.50-95.00)	82.38 (74.07-93.30)	0.407
FVC % pred. [median (IQR)]	95.72 (85.14-107.76)	96.94 (87.39-108.44)	93.49 (82.82-104.42)	0.188	88.53 (79.66-98.22)	88.85 (80.09-98.67)	85.86 (78.68-96.00)	0.418
FEV$_1$< LLN					80(31)	48(27)	32(41)	**0.036**
FEV$_1$< 80% pred.	51(20)	35(20)	16(20)	0.950	91(35)	55(31)	36(46)	**0.028**
FVC < LLN					72(28)	45(25)	27(34)	0.161
FVC < 80% pred.	47(18)	30(17)	17(22)	0.397	69(27)	44(25)	25(32)	0.273
FEV$_1$ /FVC [median (IQR)]	80.89(76.03-85.23)	80.58 (75.28-85.46)	81.60 (78.53-84.91)	0.243	80.89(76.03-85.23)	80.58 (75.28-85.46)	81.60 (78.53-84.91)	0.243
FEV$_1$ /FVC < LLN					35(14)	27(15)	8(10)	0.262
FEV$_1$ /FVC < 70%	21(8)	17(9)	4(5)	0.216	21(8)	17(9)	4(5)	0.216

FEV$_1$: forced expiratory volume in 1 second; FVC: forced vital capacity; L: litres; LLN: Lower limit of normal;
IQR: interquartile range; % pred: % predicted; *: pre-bronchodilator values, unless stated otherwise; GLI:Global lung function initiative reference values;
NHANES: National Health And Nutrition Examination Survey III reference values

Table 3.9: Summary of Health Outcomes

Health Outcome	Prevalence (%)	Males	Females	p-value
Work related Chest symptoms	80(29%)	58(31)	22(24)	0.281
Work related Ocular and nasal symptoms	57 (20%)	33(17)	24(27)	0.075
Asthma (clinical)				
Current asthma	55 (20%)	40(21)	15(17)	0.377
Asthma symptom score≥2	65 (23%)	43(23)	22(24)	0.754
COPD (clinical)	48 (17%)	29(15)	19(21)	0.233
Airway obstruction				
FEV1 < LLN (GLI)	80 (31%)	48(27)	32(41)	**0.036**
FEV1<80% predicted NHANES	51 (20%)	35(20)	16(20)	0.950
FEV1/FVC <LLN (GLI)	35 (14%)	27(15)	8(10)	0.262
FEV1/FVC<70%	21 (8%)	17(9)	4(5)	0.216
Fev1<80% and FEV1/FVC<70% (Moderate to severe obstruction)	11 (4%)	9(5)	2(3)	0.347

Current asthma: yes to any of the 3 questions: Woken up by an attack of shortness of breath in the last 12 months or Asthma attack in the past 12 months or Current use of asthma medication

Regression model development

The univariate models were developed based on known risk factors from literature
as well as the perceived risk factors in the hypothesis. The risk factors were
separately grouped into demographics and past medical history; proxies for nicotine
exposure; proxies for pesticides exposure; and proxies for biomass fuel exposure.

Multivariate models were developed using the saturated model adjusted for known
risk factors document in literature i.e. age, gender, smoking and childhood chest
infections. The biomass variable was left out in the adjustment as this was noted to
be a universal exposure for almost all workers on the farm. The selected
confounders were entered together into the model in each entry for every proxy of
exposure. This was done to allow for comparisons with findings from other studies.

Unadjusted analysis

The association between demographic characteristics and respiratory outcomes is
outlined in table 3.11a and 3.11b. Analysis is shown for both symptom-based and
spirometry- based outcomes .

Age and gender were not significantly associated with any respiratory symptom-
based outcomes. There was an increased significant association between female
gender and a low FEV_1(FEV_1<LLN) (OR 1.81, CI 1.03-3.15, p<0.05). Attaining a
secondary school education was associated with increased reporting of asthma
symptoms in both current asthma (OR 4.94, CI 1.02-23.95, p<0.05) and asthma
score≥2 (OR 3.94, CI 1.02-15.16, p<0.05) but this was not significantly associated
with spirometry based diagnoses.

There were no significant associations between smoking, alcohol use and drug use
with respiratory outcomes as outlined in table 3.11a and 3.11b.

The association between HIV infection, previous TB, past chest infections, childhood
bronchitis and respiratory outcomes is outlined below in table 3.10a and 3.10b. A
history of past chest infections during childhood showed an increased and
significant association with current asthma OR 2.86, CI 1.26 – 6.48, p<0.05), asthma

score≥2 (OR 3.64, CI 1.65-8.03, p<0.01), WRCS (OR 3.05, CI 1.40-6.66, p<0.0.01), and COPD (OR 3.52, CI 1.54-8.05, p<0.01).

For the spirometry-based outcomes past chest infections showed a significantly increased risk for FEV_1 <80% (OR 2.41, CI 1.04-5.57, p<0.05). HIV infection, previous TB, and childhood bronchitis did not show any significant association with both symptom-based and spirometry-based respiratory outcomes.

Table 3.10a: Predictors of symptom-based asthma and COPD diagnoses (unadjusted regression analysis)

Predictors n=279	Asthma score≥2	Current Asthma	COPD Symptoms	Work related ocular nasal symptoms	Work related chest symptoms
	n=65	n=55	n=48	n=57	n=80
HOST					
Age	0.99 (0.97-1.01)	0.99 (0.96 – 1.01)	1.00 (0.98-1.03)	1.01 (0.99-1.03)	0.99 (0.97-1.01)
Gender					
-Male	1.00	1.00	1.00	1.00	1.00
-Female	1.10 (0.61-1.98)	0.75 (0.39 – 1.43)	1.48 (0.78-2.81)	1.72 (0.94-3.13)	0.73 (0.41-1.29)
Smoking					
- non-smoker	1.00	1.00	1.00	1.00	1.00
- ex-smoker	2.48 (0.94-6.54)	2.62 (0.96 – 7.10)	1.30 (0.15-11.04)	1.41 (0.48-4.14)	2.25 (0.87-5.82)
- smoker	0.82 (0.39-1.70)	1.07 (0.51 – 10.32)	0.83 (0.17-4.05)	0.94 (0.45-1.98)	0.74 (0.37-1.47)
Education					
- None	1.00	1.00	1.00	1.00	1.00
- Lower primary	3.29 (0.91-11.87)	3.71 (0.81 – 17.04)	1.72 (0.53-5.57)	2.05 (0.70-5.96)	1.94 (0.66-5.64)
- Upper primary	2.45 (0.69-8.73)	3.43 (0.76 – 15.43)	1.03 (0.32-3.34)	0.91 (0.31-2.69)	2.05 (0.72-5.79)
- Secondary	**3.94 (1.02-15.16)***	**4.94 (1.02 – 23.95)***	1.81 (0.51-6.39)	1.22 (0.36-4.06)	2.93 (0.95-9.09)
Drug use	2.62 (0.87-7.85)	1.68 (0.51-5.57)	1.33 (0.36-4.97)	0.29 (0.04-2.24)	1.41 (0.46-4.34)
HIV-infected (n=228)	0.57 (0.24-1.36)	0.73 (0.30 – 1.76)	0.65 (0.25-1.65)	0.68 (0.28-1.64)	0.54 (0.25-1.21)
Alcohol use† (n=118)	2.37 (0.88-6.41)	1.82 (0.66 – 5.01)	1.70 (0.62-4.69)	0.48 (0.19-1.21)	2.50 (0.98-6.39)
History chest infection	**3.64 (1.65-8.03)****	**2.86 (1.26 – 6.48)***	**3.52 (1.54-8.05)****	1.89 (0.81-4.42)	**3.05 (1.40-6.66)****
Previous TB	0.36 (0.04-2.86)	1.79 (0.45 – 7.15)	-	0.42 (0.05-3.41)	1.69 (0.46-6.17)
Childhood bronchitis	2.74 (0.71-10.52)	3.44 (0.89 – 13.25)	1.39 (0.28-6.91)	1.12 (0.23-5.53)	0.30 (0.04-2.46)

Each entry represent a separate univariate regression between each predictor and each outcome

*= p≤0.05; **=p≤0.01; ***=p≤0.001;   † Cage Score; Define positive score ≥2/4 positive responses to CAGE questions on problem drinking

Current asthma: yes to any of the 3 questions: Woken up by an attack of shortness of breath in the last 12 months or Asthma attack in the past 12 months or Current use of asthma medication

Asthma Score category*Asthma symptom score: An asthma symptom score was computed based on the sum of answers (0=no, 1=yes) to five questions on asthma-like symptoms in the past 12 months (short of breath while wheezing, woken up with chest tightness, attack of shortness of breath at rest, attack of shortness of breath after exercise, woken up by attack of shortness of breath). Positive if yes to ≥2 questions

Table 3.10b: Predictors of spirometry-based airway obstruction diagnoses (unadjusted regression analysis)

Predictors n=258	FEV$_1$<LLN	FEV$_1$/FVC<LLN	FEV$_1$<80%[‡]	FEV$_1$/FVC<70%[‡]	Moderate/Severe Obstruction
	n=80	n=35	n=51	n=21	n=11
HOST					
Age	0.99 (0.97-1.01)	1.01 (0.98-1.04)	0.99 (0.97-1.02)	1.04 (1.00-1.07)	1.03 (0.99-1.07)
Gender					
-Male	1.00	1.00	1.00	1.00	1.00
-Female	**1.81 (1.03-3.15)***	0.62 (0.27-1.44)	1.02 (0.53-1.98)	0.50 (0.16-1.53)	0.48 (0.10-2.28)
Smoking					
- non-smoker	1.00	1.00	1.00	1.00	1.00
- ex-smoker	1.18 (0.42-3.31)	1.41 (0.38-5.24)	0.89 (0.24-3.24)	2.27 (0.59-8.72)	1.30 (0.15-11.04)
- smoker	1.25 (0.66-2.36)	1.38 (0.60-3.18)	1.52 (0.74-3.09)	0.65 (0.18-2.35)	0.83 (0.17-4.05)
Education					
- None	1.00	1.00	1.00	1.00	1.00
- Lower primary	0.72 (0.28-1.86)	0.65 (0.18-2.35)	1.12 (0.37-3.41)	0.66 (0.15-2.83)	1.03 (0.10-10.30)
- Upper primary	1.18 (0.48-2.87)	1.31 (0.41-4.20)	1.26 (0.43-3.67)	0.91 (0.23-3.51)	1.53 (0.18-13.27)
- Secondary	0.59 (0.20-1.71)	0.42 (0.09-2.05)	0.69 (0.19-2.54)	0.19 (0.02-1.89)	0.60 (0.04-10.09)
Drug use	1.72 (0.58-5.14)	1.81 (0.48-6.82)	0.66 (0.14-3.06)	1.97 (0.41-9.47)	1.8 (0.21-15.15)
HIV-infected (n=212)	1.49 (0.73-3.05)	0.87 (0.31-2.44)	1.10 (0.48-2.53)	0.82 (0.23-2.96)	1.11 (0.23-5.47)
Alcohol use† (n=110)	1.47 (0.63-3.44)	1.37 (0.40-4.70)	2.37 (0.81-6.94)	1.06 (0.18-6.06)	-
History chest infection	1.20 (0.53-2.70)	1.38 (0.49-3.90)	**2.41 (1.04-5.57)***	1.35 (0.37-4.91)	3.19 (0.80-12.77)
Previous TB	0.54 (0.11-2.63)	0.70 (0.09-5.70)	-	-	-
Childhood bronchitis	1.82 (0.48-6.97)	0.79 (0.10-6.52)	1.17 (0.23-5.79)	1.43 (0.17-12.03)	-

Each entry represent a separate univariate regression between each predictor and each outcome

*= p≤0.05; **=p≤0.01; p=≤0.001; † Cage Score; FEV$_1$: forced expiratory volume in 1 second; FVC: forced vital capacity; LLN: Lower limit of normal;

[‡]NHANES: National Health And Nutrition Examination Survey III reference values

† Cage Score; Define positive score ≥2/4 positive responses to CAGE questions on problem drinking

3.10 Pesticide exposure as a predictor of respiratory outcomes

The association between pesticide exposure and work-related symptoms, asthma and COPD symptoms, as well as lung function is outlined in table 3.11a and 3.11b. The unadjusted logistic regression models showed a significant increased association between pesticides application with current asthma (OR 2.14, CI 1.14 – 4.07, p<0.05), asthma score ≥2 (OR 2.42, CI 1.32-4.44, p<0.01), COPD (OR 2.36, CI 1.19-4.70, p<0.05), as well as ocular nasal symptoms (OR 1.88, CI 1.01-3.48, p<0.05). Pesticides exposure during spraying was associated with increased risk for asthma score (OR 2.35, CI 1.19-4.65, p<0.05,) current asthma (OR 2.76, CI 1.37 – 5.56, p<0.01) and WRONS (OR 2.60, CI 1.29-5.22, p<0.01). Participants who reported that pesticides drift had an increased risk for current asthma (OR 2.55, CI 1.01 – 6.44, p<0.05), asthma score ≥2 (OR 2.48, CI 1.01-6.11, p<0.05) and WRONS (OR 3.01, CI 1.22-7.46, p<0.05). Re-entering the field soon after spraying was also associated with increased risk for COPD 5.56 (1.30-23.79)* symptoms and decreased risk for ocular nasal symptoms (OR 0.47, CI 0.23-0.95, p<0.05). Additionally, there was a significant association showing increased risk between duration of exposure to pesticides and WRONS (OR 8.34, CI 2.73-25.54, p<0.001).

Table 3.11b shows that there was an increased risk of airflow limitation reflected in significant associations between duration of exposure to pesticides with FEV$_1$/FVC<LLN (OR 3.97, CI 1.38-11.40, p<0.05), FEV$_1$/FVC<70% (OR 3.89, CI 1.30-11.36, p<0.05), and moderate to severe airway obstruction (OR 5.12, CI 1.53-17.16, p<0.01). Additionally, using pesticides at home was significantly associated with a decreased risk for having a lower lung ratio (FEV$_1$/FVC<LLN) (table 3.12b)..

3.11 Nicotine exposure as a predictor of respiratory outcomes

The association between nicotine exposure and work related symptoms, asthma and COPD symptoms, as well as lung function is outlined in table 3.11a and 3.11b. The unadjusted logistic regression models show that having reported a history of a GTS episode was significantly associated with all symptom-based diagnoses (OR ranging from 2.12 to 6.93, p<0.05 to p<001).

Certain tasks like sowing and transplanting were significantly associated with all respiratory symptoms (OR ranging from 2.48 to 6.26, p<0.001 to p<0.05). Harvesting was significantly associated with WRCS (OR 2.57, CI 1.37-4.83, p<0.01), WRONS (OR 7.79, CI 3.96-15.30, p<0.001), COPD symptoms (OR 2.23, CI 1.09-4.57, p<0.05), Current asthma (OR 2.03 CI 1.01 – 4.06, p<0.05), but not significantly with asthma score. Curing showed an increased significant strong association with WRONS (OR 18.10 CI 7.49-43.72, p<0.001) only.

There were no significant associations between nicotine exposure variables and lung function indices.

Table 3.11a: Predictors of symptom-based asthma and COPD diagnoses (unadjusted regression analysis) related to Exposures

	Asthma score≥2	Current Asthma	COPD Symptoms	Work related ocular nasal symptoms	Work related chest symptoms
Predictors n=279	n=65	n=55	n=48	n=57	n=80
Nicotine Exposure					
Previous GTS episode	**2.80 (1.58-4.94)*****	**3.03 (1.65 – 5.54)*****	**2.12 (1.13-3.98)***	**5.4 (2.89-10.09)*****	**3.82 (2.22-6.59)*****
GTS episode in past year	**3.41 (1.88-6.16)*****	**3.73 (2.01 – 6.94)*****	**2.68 (1.40-5.12)****	**6.93 (3.67-13.05)*****	**3.30 (1.87-5.80)*****
Activities related to GTS					
- Sowing	**3.92 (1.76-8.75)****	**5.12 (2.27 – 11.55)*****	**5.35 (2.35-12.19)*****	**4.84 (2.15-10.88)*****	**2.80 (1.27-6.19)***
- Transplanting	**4.18 (1.75-10.00)****	**2.93 (1.20 – 7.19)***	**5.43 (2.23-13.20)*****	**6.26 (2.58-15.19)*****	**2.48 (1.05-5.89)***
- Harvesting	1.94 (1.00-3.78)	**2.03 (1.01 – 4.06)***	**2.23 (1.09-4.57)***	**7.79 (3.96-15.30)*****	**2.57 (1.37-4.83)****
- Curing	1.98 (0.89-4.38)	2.15 (0.95 – 4.87)	1.81 (0.76-4.33)	**18.10 (7.49-43.72)*****	1.67 (0.77-3.63)
Other	**3.98 (1.82-8.68)****	**3.19 (1.43 – 7.11)****	1.54 (0.62-3.84)	0.76 (0.28-2.08)	**4.52 (2.06-9.92)*****
Pesticide Exposure (279)					
Workplace Pesticides application	**2.42 (1.32-4.44)****	**2.15 (1.14 – 4.07)***	**2.36 (1.19-4.70)***	**1.88 (1.01-3.48)***	1.63 (0.95-2.79)
-Duration in Hrs/day (158)	1.01 (0.71-1.42)	0.84 (0.46 – 1.54)	1.12 (0.81-1.56)	**8.34 (2.73-25.54)*****	0.97 (0.68-1.39)
Work near pesticide sprayers	1.15 (0.62-2.16)	1.07 (0.55 – 2.06)	1.88 (0.87-4.10)	0.67 (0.36-1.24)	1.06 (0.59-1.89)
Environmental					
Exposure during spraying	**2.35 (1.19-4.65)***	**2.76 (1.37 – 5.56)****	1.47 (0.67-3.23)	**2.60 (1.29-5.22)****	1.65 (0.84-3.21)
Pesticide drift	**2.48 (1.01-6.11)***	**2.55 (1.01 – 6.44)***	1.46 (0.51-4.18)	**3.01 (1.22-7.46)***	1.81 (0.74-4.43)
Field re-entry after spraying	2.33 (0.94-5.77)	1.49 (0.63 – 3.54)	**5.56 (1.30-23.79)***	**0.47 (0.23-0.95)***	1.21 (0.59-2.47)
Home use of pesticides)	1.49 (0.85-2.61)	1.31 (0.73 – 2.38)	1.30 (0.69-2.43)	0.64 (0.36-1.15)	0.95 (0.57-1.60)

Each entry represent a separate univariate regression between each predictor and each outcome
*= p≤0.05; **=p≤0.01; ***=p≤0.001;
Current asthma: yes to any of the 3 questions: Woken up by an attack of shortness of breath in the last 12 months or Asthma attack in the past 12 months or Current use of asthma medication
Asthma Score category*Asthma symptom score: An asthma symptom score was computed based on the sum of answers (0=no, 1=yes) to five questions on asthma-like symptoms in the past 12 months (short of breath while wheezing, woken up with chest tightness, attack of shortness of breath at rest, attack of shortness of breath after exercise, woken up by attack of shortness of breath). Positive if yes to ≥2 questions
WRON symptoms: work related nasal-ocular symptoms; WRC symptoms: work related chest symptoms

Table 3.11b: Predictors of spirometry-based airway obstruction diagnoses (unadjusted regression analysis) related to Exposures

	FEV_1<LLN	FEV_1/FVC<LLN	FEV_1<80%[‡]	FEV_1/FVC<70%[‡]	Moderate/Severe Obstruction
Predictors n=258	n=80	n=35	n=51	n=21	n=11
Nicotine Exposure					
Previous GTS episode	0.93 (0.53-1.62)	0.97 (0.46-2.05)	0.58 (0.29-1.15)	0.93 (0.36-2.39)	0.69 (0.18-2.67)
GTS episode in past year	0.87 (0.47-1.60)	1.19 (0.53-2.63)	0.65 (0.30-1.40)	1.51 (0.58-3.92)	1.10 (0.28-4.26)
Activities related to GTS					
- Sowing	0.47 (0.17-1.30)	0.48 (0.11-2.12)	0.48 (0.14-165)	0.41 (0.52-3.15)	0.85 (0.10-6.91)
- Transplanting	0.50 (0.16-1.53)	0.30 (0.04-2.30)	0.40 (0.09-1.79)	0.54 (0.07-4.26)	1.14 (0.14-9.32)
- Harvesting	0.92 (0.45-1.87)	0.59 (0.20-1.77)	0.59 (0.24-1.49)	0.80 (0.22-2.83)	0.47 (0.06-3.80)
- Curing	1.35 (0.59-3.10)	1.12 (0.36-3.46)	0.91 (0.33-2.54)	0.89 (0.20-4.06)	0.85 (0.10-6.91)
- Other	1.06 (0.46-2.46)	2.40 (0.94-6.17)	0.65 (0.21-1.96)	2.09 (0.65-6.72)	0.81 (0.10-6.61)
Pesticide Exposure					
Pesticides application	0.77 (0.45-1.30)	0.82 (0.40-1.66)	1.05 (0.57-1.96)	0.70 (0.29-1.71)	0.65 (0.19-2.18)
Duration of exposure(Hrs/day)(144)	1.74 (0.72-4.21)	**3.97 (1.38-11.40)***	1.98 (0.80-4.86)	**3.89 (1.33-11.36)***	**5.12 (1.53-17.16)****
Work near pesticide sprayers	0.79 (0.44-1.41)	0.96 (0.44-2.12)	1.52 (0.73-3.16)	0.96 (0.36-2.59)	0.66 (0.19-2.34)
Exposure during spraying	1.14 (0.56-2.30)	0.84 (0.31-2.30)	0.95 (0.41-2.19)	0.85 (0.24-3.01)	1.15 (0.24-5.52)
Pesticide drift	1.54 (0.60-3.92)	1.67 (0.52-5.32)	0.70 (0.20-2.48)	2.16 (0.58-8.06)	2.83 (0.57-14.08)
Field re-entry after spraying	0.96 (0.47-1.97)	0.72 (0.29-1.78)	1.02 (0.44-2.36)	0.57 (0.20-1.66)	0.84 (0.18-4.06)
Home use of pesticides	0.79 (0.47-1.35)	**0.42 (0.20-0.88)***	0.92 (0.50-1.69)	0.52 (0.21-1.31)	0.50 (0.14-1.74)

Each entry represent a separate univariate regression between each predictor and each outcome
*= p≤0.05; **=p≤0.01; ***=p≤0.001; FEV_1: forced expiratory volume in 1 second; FVC: forced vital capacity; LLN: Lower limit of normal;
[‡]NHANES: National Health And Nutrition Examination Survey III reference values

3.12 Biomass exposure as a predictor of respiratory outcomes

The association between biomass exposure and work- related symptoms, asthma
and COPD symptoms, as well as lung function is outlined in table 3.12a. The logistic
regression models (unadjusted) showed an increased significant association
between cooking tasks using biomass fuel with work related nasal-ocular symptoms
(OR 2.80, CI 1.14-6.88, p≤0.05) and a protective effect with WRCS (OR 0.44, CI
0.22-0.80, P<0.01).

Logistic regression models of lung function indices indicated an increased
association between biomass exposure at work and airflow limitation as reflected in
FEV_1<80% of predicted (OR 2.20, CI 1.08-4.46, p<0.05).

Table 3.12a: Predictors of symptom-based asthma and COPD diagnoses (unadjusted regression analysis) related to Biomass Exposure

	Asthma score≥2	Current Asthma	COPD Symptoms	Work related nasal ocular symptoms	Work related chest symptoms
Predictors n=279	n=65	n=55	n=48	n=57	n=80
Biomass Fuel					
Exposure to biomass fuel	0.79 (0.36-1.74)	1.31 (0.52-3.32)	1.38 (0.51-3.75)	3.26 (0.96-11.01)	0.62 (0.30-1.27)
Biomass fuel source					
-Home	0.90 (0.51-1.59)	1.31 (0.72 – 2.37)	1.09 (0.58-2.05)	1.01 (0.56-1.82)	1.64 (0.85-3.14)
- Work	1.27 (0.63-2.59)	0.78 (0.34 – 1.78)	1.56 (0.73-3.33)	0.88 (0.40-1.94)	0.77 (0.45-1.32)
Tasks associated with exposure					
-cooking	0.59 (0.31-1.11)	1.15 (0.55-2.39)	1.49 (0.66-3.78)	**2.80 (1.14-6.88)***	**0.44 (0.22-0.80)****
-curing tobacco	0.98 (0.56-1.72)	0.84 (0.46-1.53)	1.02 (0.54-1.91)	1.46 (0.82-2.62)	0.95 (0.56-1.61)
-smoking tobacco	0.65 (0.14-3.03)	0.81 (0.17-3.80)	0.96 (0.23-4.53)	1.31 (0.34-5.02)	1.26 (0.37-4.30)
Duration of exposure					
Hours per day (n=241)	0.90 (0.81-1.01)	0.83 (0.72-0.95)	1.05 (0.95-1.16)	0.92 (0.83-1.03)	0.93 (0.84-1.02)

Each entry represent a separate univariate regression between each predictor and each outcome
*= p≤0.05; **=p≤0.01; ***=p≤0.001;
ECRHS Definition of asthma:
Asthma Score category*Asthma symptom score: An asthma symptom score was computed based on the sum of answers (0=no, 1=yes) to five questions on asthma-like symptoms in the past 12 months (short of breath while wheezing, woken up with chest tightness, attack of shortness of breath at rest, attack of shortness of breath after exercise, woken up by attack of shortness of breath). Positive if yes to ≥2 questions
WRON symptoms: work related nasal-ocular symptoms; WRC symptoms: work related chest symptoms

Table 3.12b: Predictors of spirometry-based airway obstruction diagnoses (unadjusted regression analysis) related to biomass exposures

	FEV_1<LLN	FEV_1/FVC<LLN	FEV_1<80%[‡]	FEV_1/FVC<70%[‡]	Moderate/Severe Obstruction
Predictors n= 258	n=80	n=35	n=51	n=21	n=11
Biomass Fuel					
Exposure to biomass fuel	0.84 (0.38-1.83)	0.64 (0.24-1.68)	1.08 (0.42-2.77)	0.57 (0.18-1.81)	1.44 (0.18-11.60)
Biomass fuel source					
-Home	0.92 (0.54-1.57)	0.93 (0.45-1.93)	0.65 (0.34-1.24)	0.86 (0.34-2.14)	0.80 (0.23-2.80)
- Work	1.43 (0.74-2.76)	1.63 (0.71-3.76)	**2.20 (1.08-4.46)***	1.41 (0.49-4.06)	2.64 (0.74-9.40)
Tasks associated with exposure					
-cooking	1.04 (0.55-1.98)	0.47 (0.22-1.02)	1.17 (0.55-2.52)	0.41 (0.16-1.05)	0.47 (0.13-1.66)
-curing tobacco	1.03 (0.60-1.74)	0.81 (0.39-1.66)	1.52 (0.82-2.81)	0.93 (0.38-2.28)	1.52 (0.45-5.11)
-smoking tobacco	1.12 (0.33-3.83)	Uncalculable	1.38 (0.36-5.27)	Uncalculable	Uncalculable
Duration of exposure					
- Hours per day (n=225)	1.03 (0.94-1.12)	1.07 (0.95-1.20)	1.10 (1.00-1.21)	1.10 (0.96-1.27)	1.10 (0.92-1.31)

Each entry represent a separate univariate regression between each predictor and each outcome
*= p≤0.05; **=p≤0.01; ***=p≤0.001;
FEV_1: forced expiratory volume in 1 second; FVC: forced vital capacity; LLN: Lower limit of normal;
[‡]NHANES: National Health And Nutrition Examination Survey III reference values

A multivariate model of respiratory symptoms adjusted for age, gender, smoking
status, and childhood respiratory infections is shown in table 3.13a below. Proxies
for nicotine exposure, were used i.e. previous GTS episodes. Two activities (sowing
and transplanting) associated with GTS episode showed a significant association
with all symptom-based respiratory outcomes (OR 1.78-7.26, p<0.05 to p<0.001).
Harvesting was significantly associated with increased odds of all symptom-based
outcomes (OR 1.93-8.81, p<0.05 to p<0.001) except for current asthma. Curing was
associated with current asthma (OR 2.40, CI 1.01-5.71, p<0.05) and work-related
nasal-ocular symptoms (OR 22.45, CI 8.74-57.68, p<0.001).

Pesticide application showed an increased association with all symptom-based
respiratory outcomes (OR 1.96-2.62, p>0.01 to p<0.05) except WRCS. Exposure
during spraying was significantly associated with increased odds of current asthma
(OR 2.57, CI 1.22-5.40, p<0.05), asthma score (OR 2.09, CI 1.01-4.31, p<0.05),
WRONS (OR 2.43, CI 1.17-5.04, p<0.05). Pesticide drift was significantly associated
with increased odds of current asthma (OR 2.62, CI 1.01-6.86, p<0.05). Re-entry of
fields after spraying showed an increased significant association with COPD
symptoms (OR 5.22, CI 1.20-22.75, p<0.05) and protective against ocular nasal
symptoms (OR 0.45, CI 0.22-0.92, p<0.05) while number of hours of exposure to
pesticides showed an increased significant association with WRONS (OR 9.50, CI
2.97-30.34, p<0.001).

Multivariate model for spirometry-based outcomes after adjusting for age, gender,
smoking, and childhood infections is shown in Table 3.13b. all proxies for nicotine
exposure did not show any significant associations with the outcomes. Most proxies
for pesticide exposure did not show any significant association with respiratory
outcomes except for duration of pesticide exposure which showed increased
significant association with FEV1/FVC<LLN (OR 5.11, CI 1.57-16.66, p<0.01),
FEV1/FVC<70% (OR 4.58, CI 1.17-17.98, p<0.05), and moderate to severe airway
obstruction (OR 13.25, CI 1.69-103.93, p<0.05).

Table 3.13a: Multivariate analysis of predictors of symptom-based asthma and COPD diagnoses†

	Asthma score≥2	Current Asthma	COPD Symptoms	WR Nasal-ocular symptoms	WR chest symptoms
	n=65	n=55	n=48	n=57	n=80
Nicotine Exposure (n=279)			OR (95% CI)		
Previous GTS episode	2.68 (1.48-4.83)**	2.89 (1.55-5.39)**	2.19 (1.12-4.26)*	5.94 (3.10-11.40)***	3.64 (2.08-6.37)***
GTS episode in past year	3.28 (1.76-6.13)***	3.58 (1.87-6.85)***	3.03 (1.49-6.19)**	9.14 (4.51-18.51)***	3.02 (1.68-5.45)***
Activities related to GTS					
- Sowing	3.78 (1.62-8.85)**	4.93 (2.10-11.55)***	7.26 (2.86-18.41)***	5.74 (2.43-13.56)***	2.49 (1.09-5.70)*
- Transplanting	3.80 (1.52-9.45)**	2.65 (1.04-6.76)*	5.43 (2.08-14.21)**	6.18 (2.49-15.35)***	2.23 (0.91-5.50)
- Harvesting	1.93 (0.96-3.87)	2.01 (0.98-4.13)	2.40 (1.12-5.15)*	8.81 (4.33-17.91)***	2.65 (1.37-5.11)**
- Curing	2.11 (0.91-4.88)	2.40 (1.01-5.71)*	2.09 (0.81-5.40)	22.45 (8.74-57.68)***	1.78 (0.79-4.02)
- Other	3.84 (1.68-8.75)**	2.92 (1.24-6.72)*	1.34 (0.49-3.66)	0.70 (0.24-2.00)	4.07 (1.81-9.17)**
Pesticide Exposure (n=279)					
Pesticide application	2.35 (1.24-4.44)*	2.05 (1.05-3.99)*	2.62 (1.25-5.51)*	1.96 (1.03-3.71)*	1.50 (0.85-2.62)
Exposure during spraying	2.09 (1.01-4.31)*	2.57 (1.22-5.40)*	1.05 (0.45-2.49)	2.43 (1.17-5.04)*	1.54 (0.75-3.13)
Pesticide drift	2.43 (0.96-6.17)	2.62 (1.00-6.86)*	1.42 (0.47-4.28)	3.00 (1.18-7.62)*	1.81 (0.72-4.58)
Field re-entry after spraying	2.13 (0.85-5.35)	1.31 (0.55-3.16)	5.22 (1.20-22.75)*	0.45 (0.22-0.92)*	1.09 (0.53-2.27)
Duration of exposure (Hrs/day)	1.06 (0.75-1.49)	0.92 (0.54-1.58)	1.20 (0.86-1.68)	9.50 (2.97-30.34)***	1.02 (0.72-1.45)

*= p≤0.05; **=p≤0.01; ***=p≤0.001;

Current asthma: defined as either having shortness of breath in the past 12 months or an asthma attack in the past 12 months or current use of asthma medication

Asthma Score category*Asthma symptom score: An asthma symptom score was computed based on the sum of answers (0=no, 1=yes) to five questions on asthma-like symptoms in the past 12 months (short of breath while wheezing, woken up with chest tightness, attack of shortness of breath at rest, attack of shortness of breath after exercise, woken up by attack of shortness of breath). Positive if yes to ≥2 questions

WRON symptoms: work related nasal-ocular symptoms; WRC symptoms: work related chest symptoms

† Each estimate based on individual regression models that have been adjusted for age, gender smoking and childhood chest infections

Table 3.13b: Multivariate analysis of predictors of spirometry-based airway obstruction diagnoses†

Predictors n= 258	FEV_1<LLN	FEV_1/FVC<LLN	FEV_1<80%[‡]	FEV_1/FVC<70%[‡]	Moderate/Severe Obstruction
	n=80	n=35	n=51	n=21	n=11
Nicotine Exposure (n=279)		OR (95% CI)			
Previous GTS episode	0.95 (0.54-1.68)	0.95 (0.44-2.04)	0.55 (0.27-1.12)	0.87 (0.32-2.33)	0.58 (0.14-2.37)
GTS episode in past year	0.89 (0.47-1.67)	1.20 (0.53-2.72)	0.64 (0.29-1.39)	1.41 (0.52-3.88)	0.95 (0.22-4.00)
Activities related to GTS					
- Sowing	0.45 (0.16-1.27)	0.48 (0.11-2.17)	0.43 (0.12-1.54)	0.42 (0.05-3.38)	0.81 (0.09-7.15)
- Transplanting	0.45 (0.14-1.42)	0.28 (0.04-2.22)	0.34 (0.07-1.55)	0.52 (0.06-4.32)	0.96 (0.11-8.51)
- Harvesting	0.89 (0.43-1.83)	0.59 (0.20-1.79)	0.58 (0.23-1.49)	0.80 (0.22-2.93)	0.49 (0.06-4.02)
- Curing	1.34 (0.58-3.13)	1.23 (0.39-3.82)	1.00 (0.34-2.83)	0.87 (0.18-4.13)	0.91 (0.11-7.76)
- Other	1.19 (0.50-2.83)	2.24 (0.85-5.91)	0.61 (0.19-1.90)	1.66 (0.48-5.74)	0.49 (0.05-4.56)
Pesticides					
Pesticide application	0.74 (0.43-1.28)	0.79 (0.38-1.66)	0.92 (0.48-1.75)	0.77 (0.30-1.97)	0.56 (0.15-2.06)
Exposure during spraying	0.96 (0.46-2.01)	0.81 (0.28-2.34)	0.72 (0.29-1.76)	1.05 (0.28-4.00)	1.12 (0.21-6.08)
Pesticide drift	1.39 (0.54-3.60)	1.91 (0.58-6.23)	0.69 (0.19-2.52)	2.84 (0.71-11.38)	4.01 (0.74-21.86)
Field re-entry after spraying	0.91 (0.43-1.89)	0.71 (0.28-1.79)	0.94 (0.40-2.21)	0.65 (0.21-1.97)	0.91 (0.18-4.60)
Duration of exposure (Hrs/day)	1.97 (0.80-4.84)	**5.11 (1.57-16.66)****	2.41 (0.95-6.11)	**4.58 (1.17-17.98)***	**13.25 (1.69-103.93)***

*= p≤0.05; **=p≤0.01; ***=p≤0.001;
FEV_1: forced expiratory volume in 1 second; FVC: forced vital capacity; LLN: Lower limit of normal;
[‡]NHANES: National Health And Nutrition Examination Survey III reference values
† Each estimate based on individual regression models that have been adjusted for age, gender, smoking and childhood chest infections

CHAPTER 4: DISCUSSION

This study reveals that tobacco farmers in this setting are predominantly young adults most of whom are educated to the primary level with a mean employment duration of 7.3 years. These farmers are more exposed to risky social behaviors such as current alcohol consumption (42%) and current smoking (20%) compared to the national average of 17.3% and 11% respectively[80]. A study among urban dwellers in Malawi revealed a lower prevalence of ever smoking of 10% compared to 27% in our study[6]. One Brazilian study among tobacco farmers reported a comparable prevalence of smokers among tobacco farmers of 17% though another Brazilian study reported a high prevalence of 33%[68,13]. Lopes investigated factors associated with heavy drinking among 2469 randomly selected tobacco farmers[81]. Their findings showed that high risk and heavy drinking were associated with male gender, having no partner, being an employee, frequency of pesticide use in both males and females. Among males, other risk factors for drinking were smoking (PR 1.46, CI 1.22-1.73), higher working hours (>12) (PR 1.81, CI 1.19-2.74), crop loss (PR 1.24, CI 1.06-1.45), having a loan (PR 1.62, CI 1.24-2.13). While the factors above could be relevant to this study, a higher prevalence of smoking and alcohol in this rural population may signify a lack of health information related to healthier lifestyles among these rural farmers compared other parts of the country where health information is readily available through various media portals. The experience showed that the farms were located in very remote and hard to reach areas where it was difficult to access phone networks. It was also noted that these farms did not have any particular workplace health programs or policies in place.

There was an observation of a very high prevalence of HIV infection (16%) in this particular population which is double the national average of 8%. The Demographic and Health survey 2015-2016 reported that HIV prevalence in Malawi is high in urban settings with an average of 14.6% compared to rural areas at 7.4%[82]. Another study observing the trends in HIV prevalence in Northern Malawi demonstrated a higher HIV prevalence among women closer to the roads than those in remote areas among those tested at antenatal clinics[83]. There was a higher HIV prevalence in our sample despite the fact that this was a rural setting. It could be speculated that the daily earning capacity among the seasonal workers and larger labor force in these estates put these workers at a particular social risk in their environment similar to that observed in higher income populations.

Previous chest infections in childhood were significantly associated with chest diagnoses such as asthma, COPD, and work- related chest symptoms but not ocular nasal symptoms. History of chest infection is a documented risk factor for obstructive lung diseases[84]. Although the types of past infections were not documented in this study, in general terms, infections are associated with activation of both immune-mediated and irritant mechanisms likely to affect those affected making their airways hyper-responsive to other stimuli[85].

This study demonstrates a higher prevalence of obstructive lung diseases (asthma and chronic bronchitis) among tobacco farmers in Malawi compared to other studies. The findings in other studies measuring individual respiratory symptoms such as wheezes among tobacco farmers found lower prevalence of 11%[13] and 16%[86]. Other symptoms in this study, such as shortness of breath (30%), were comparable to findings by Gosh and others (20%)[87] and higher than a study by Van Minh (24.3%)[37]. The strength of this study is the use of the standardized symptoms definitions of asthma and chronic bronchitis which other studies among tobacco farmers did not demonstrate. This enables us to establish that obstructive lung diseases are more prevalent among tobacco farm workers than previously thought.

One unique feature of this particular study is the characteristic higher prevalence of work-related chest symptoms compared to upper airway symptoms. Usually, airborne workplace respiratory hazards such as dust reach the upper airways first in higher concentrations. Due to immune mechanisms in the respiratory tract the concentration is gradually reduced down the tract as more particles get trapped before they descend to the lower respiratory tract. Thus, one would expect more and early symptoms to be manifested on the upper side of the respiratory tract than otherwise. However, this is not the pattern of respiratory symptoms demonstrated in this study. There could be possible explanations for this particular pattern. Firstly, it could be that the hazard responsible for these respiratory effects reaches the respiratory system through some other route other than the respiratory system. The possible route could be dermal, in case of both nicotine and pesticides. This makes it possible for the hazard to evade the natural airway protective mechanism and reach any part of the body including the lungs in somewhat different concentrations and exert its effects there. This is likely to happen in this population especially considering the low prevalence of those using personal protective equipment. Another explanation could be that the characteristics of the upper airways make it more resilient to this particular hazard encountered by tobacco farmers than does the lower respiratory tract. Thirdly, a hazard with very small particle sizes in the respirable ranges or those in gaseous forms are likely to reach the lower parts of the respiratory system in rather higher concentrations. In the context of the delicate nature of that part of the respiratory tract an exposed individual may experience the adverse effects quicker than otherwise.

There was a higher prevalence (20%) of spirometry- based airway obstruction among rural based tobacco farmers demonstrated in this study compared to the urban dwellers (3.6%) using similar reference values (NHANES III)[6]. Moderate to severe obstruction (sub-optimal FEV1 and FEV1/FVC) was higher among the tobacco farmers than the urban dwellers. This finding points to the significant role that occupational exposures in the tobacco farms may have on respiratory health outcomes. The association between tobacco farming and airway limitations observed through spirometry has been previously described[88,87]. While there was comparable prevalence of other important exposures such as using biomass fuel between the two populations the notable exposure differences were occupation and high smoking prevalence. Urban dwellers do not usually engage in commercial farm activities since most farms are located in the remote country sides. The tobacco farmers also demonstrated a higher prevalence of obstruction when calculations were based on the GLI reference equation FEV1<Lower Limit of Normal (LLN), 31%. Use of spirometry equations in interpreting spirometry results should seriously consider the racial or ethnic differences. While the NHANES reference equations applied in this study are derived from multiple races which include African Americans the GLI equations were mainly based on the European population leading to overestimation of abnormalities[89,90]. Despite the limitations, NHANES references were used to provide a basis of comparison with other studies in Malawi which were conducted based on these references. The GLI equation was used to generate a distribution of

our sample on which to base our lower limit values. The discrepancies observed with usage of GLI in Africa has prompted recommendations to incorporate African data in these equations.

In this study, GTS was used as proxy measure for nicotine exposure. GTS was defined as having any of the four symptoms (headache, dizziness, nausea, and vomiting) and was noted in 26% of the participants in the previous year. This was relatively higher than one of the Brazilian studies which needed at least 2 symptoms to define GTS in which the prevalence was 11%[13]. When the definition was modified to align with the Brazilian study, the prevalence dropped to 14% which is still higher but comparable. Another Brazilian study documented a much higher prevalence of GTS reaching up to 67% of the participants despite being a smaller sample size of 100 conveniently selected participants subjecting it to selection bias[68]. Other studies have reported rather higher prevalence based on more inclusive definitions of the condition such as gastrointestinal and respiratory symptoms[87].

Farmers reported an average of three GTS episodes in a year and reported most of the symptoms appearing on the same day of exposure. This is comparable to the study by Fiori which reported a majority have 1 to 5 GTS episodes within a year[13]. Main tasks associated with GTS symptoms were harvesting followed by curing. Harvesting tobacco has been documented as the commonest source of nicotine exposure through the dermal route among tobacco farmers. In this setting tobacco harvesters perform their tasks without protective equipment making them susceptible to nicotine absorption through the skin. In Malawi, tobacco is harvested in December and January and usually in the morning hours. These months are the wettest months in the calendar in terms of rain fall. Harvesting in the morning, subjects the farmers to other forms of moist conditions such as morning dew. All these conditions promote nicotine absorption and subsequent toxicity predisposing to GTS.

Flue-curing involved collecting green tobacco leaves soon after harvesting and hanging them in curing barns by tying them. While harvesting was done by a majority of the workers, curing was done by a selected few who were trained in the processes. Since these estates produce flue-cured tobacco, it meant that these selected individuals had to touch every tobacco leaf that was harvested by hanging them to the barns. In the early stages of harvesting the same workers were also involved in harvesting. Even though harvesting involved larger numbers of workers in general it could be postulated that individuals involved in curing in these estates were likely to succumb to the dose-dependent effects of nicotine exposure. A comparable number of participants reported tasks such as sowing as being responsible for their symptoms. While this relationship is not documented, sowing is generally associated with rigorous use of pesticides and it is the peak stage of pesticides application during tobacco cultivation. It is possible that the symptoms reported could be as a result of pesticide poisoning as reported in other studies[91,92].

GTS was significantly associated with an increase of all symptom based respiratory outcomes both independently and after adjusting for age, sex, smoking, and childhood infections. Fiori et al demonstrated a relationship between number of GTS episodes and occurrence of wheeze among tobacco farmers[13]. Although their study did not have extensive evaluation of the respiratory symptoms, wheezing was used as a proxy for asthma. In this study, GTS was associated with both definitions of asthma as well as COPD. This finding adds value to the existing evidence indicating that beyond wheezing nicotine exposure is also associated with other types of chronic respiratory symptoms signifying chronic bronchitis. Furthermore, the symptoms of GTS were associated with both work-related upper and lower respiratory symptoms. This might indicate the role of nicotine as an occupational hazard in the occurrence of these symptoms.

Following absorption of nicotine including dermal means, it enters into the blood stream where only less than 5% is bound to plasm proteins. The rest is extensively distributed to body tissues with highest affinity for the brain, liver, kidney, spleen and the lungs[22]. An in vitro study on human airway cell culture exposure to nicotine revealed its effects on the viscosity of airway mucins[57]. Mucins exposed to nicotine were aggregated and less hydrated causing them to be thicker. The investigator postulated that this mechanism could explain why smokers usually have thicker airway secretions. The high affinity of lung cells to nicotine may lead to a considerable exposure of the cells to similar effects in vivo even though this has not been documented. In vivo nicotine has been demonstrated to influence the respiratory system directly or indirectly through the nervous system leading to bronchoconstriction and excess mucus production[58]. Studies on respiratory health effects of nicotine exposure through tobacco smoke show that nicotine plays a role in development of emphysema by decreasing elastin in the alveolar parenchyma and increased alveolar volume which leads to development of COPD. Its effects on the autonomic nervous system through vagal reflexes have been shown to cause bronchoconstriction[21].

Three main activities (sowing, transplanting, and harvesting) were significantly associated with asthma, COPD, work related upper and lower respiratory symptoms in our multivariate analysis. Curing was associated with all respiratory outcomes except work related chest symptoms. While transplanting, harvesting and curing are involved with touching the fresh tobacco plant or leaves, sowing does not involve touching the tobacco plant. However, during sowing farmers are extensively exposed to tobacco pesticides used to sterilize the nurseries. The association observed in this task with GTS symptoms could be non-specifically linked to chemical exposure. Fiori and others found a relationship between lifting tobacco sticks to the curing barns and wheezing[13]. Nevertheless, harvesting and curing which are associated with high nicotine exposure have been linked with development of respiratory symptoms in our study.

There was a higher prevalence of farmers in this study who reported contact with pesticides at work compared to other documented studies among tobacco farmers[13], with the exception of one other study which documented a much higher proportion (97%) of farm workers contacting pesticides[68]. Of particular interest is the fact that only less than half of the farmers who reported to work with pesticides indicated pesticides handling as their job title. This signifies a possible danger in pesticide exposure to individuals who are not trained to handle pesticides. Another key finding was that several pesticides that were reported as being used by participants were different from the list of recommended pesticides for use by the Tobacco Commission in the country[26]. For example, some of the pesticides reported in this study were banned for use among tobacco farmers based on their updated guidelines which considers both resistance as well environmental effects. AChE inhibitors (including organophosphates) constituted the commonly used group of pesticides. Several other factors put these participants at an increased risk of pesticide exposure including: inadequate use of personal protective equipment by sprayers and other farm workers; a very high percentage (83%) reported entering fields soon after spraying implying a much greater proportion are exposed to pesticides. It was noted that as much as half of the participants used pesticides at home for their own gardens and grain storage. The commonest used pesticide at participants' homes were pirimiphos-methyl which is also an AChE inhibitor and have similar effects as organophosphates used in the tobacco fields. The proportion of farmers using AChE inhibitors at home is twice as much as those using the chemicals in the field. This finding demonstrates that workplace data alone may underestimate the magnitude of exposure and their health effects among these participants.

This study has documented the major groups of pesticides involved in the tobacco cultivation process in Malawi and their proportion of use. Of note is that most of the listed pesticides have been independently associated with adverse respiratory effects among farmers through various mechanisms[48]. The effect of concurrent use of these groups of pesticides on the health outcomes is uncertain.

The study revealed an association between pesticides exposure and asthma definitions, chronic bronchitis, as well as work related ocular nasal symptoms but not work- related chest symptoms. Wheeze was shown to be associated with exposure to pesticides in Agriculture Health Study among commercial pesticide applicators by Hoppin[39]. After adjusting for confounders organophosphates remained significantly associated with wheeze (OR 2.72, 95 percent CI: 1.54, 4.81). The fact that AChE inhibitors were more prevalent in our study than any other pesticides may explain the similar trends in this study. A study in Brazil among agricultural health workers showed an increased association between pesticides (generally) and adult onset asthma (OR = 1.54, 95% CI: 1.04–2.58)[30] while a Canadian study on male farmers showed an association between self-reported asthma and carbamate (AChE inhibitor) pesticides (OR = 1.8, 95% CI: 1.1–3.1)[93].

Several studies have shown the role of pesticide exposure in airway symptoms including both atopic and non-atopic asthma. Hoppin demonstrated that several pesticides were associated with atopic asthma while some like DDT were associated with non-atopic asthma[39]. A study among French farmers found an increased association between pesticide exposure and allergic asthma (OR 1.97, CI 1.43–2.73) than non-allergic asthma (OR 1.24, CI 0.88–1.76)[94]. The authors postulated that the allergic mechanisms could be through indirect effects of pesticides on the immune system such as Th1 and Th2. Both animal and human studies of AChE exposure through organophosphates and organochlorides demonstrate Th1 suppression with concurrent increase in Th2 suggesting type 1 reactions[95]. A study by Mwanga demonstrated an association between organophosphates and pyrethroids with probable allergic asthma (FeNO>50ppb) through Th2 and non-Th2 mechanisms[40]. Another study by Ndlovu exhibited a positive associationbetween AChE suppression due to pesticide exposure and possible allergic asthma (FeNO>25ppb)[41]. In the same study several proxies for pesticide exposure were independently associated with a higher asthma score. Low AChE (OR 1.93, CI 1.09-3.44), Pesticide drift (OR 2.03, CI 1.38-2.98), number of pesticides spraying days (OR 1.01, CI 1.00-1.01) were significantly associated with increased asthma score. The present study shows the significance of duration of exposure as a predictor of dose. The findings showed an increased though non-significant relationship between duration of pesticide use and asthma score, COPD, and work-related chest symptoms. The isolated stronger and significant increased association observed between the duration of exposure and ocular nasal symptoms could be due to the acute effects occurring during spraying. Duration of exposure to pesticides is documented as an important predictor of toxicity[28]. These relationships reported in the above studies are in agreement with the existent associations between pesticide exposure proxies and asthma outcomes in our study.

It has been observed in animal studies (guinea pigs) that AChE inhibitor pesticides such as organophosphates induce airway hyperactivity at doses lower than those that show effects of AChE inhibition[96]. This has been shown to occur through neural and inflammatory pathways. Organophosphates either induce airways hyperactivity by potentiating M3 airway smooth muscle receptors or by blocking autoinhibitory M2 receptors on airway parasympathetic nerves. Low level organophosphates were also observed to enhance immune responses to other chemical allergens and to exacerbate eosinophilia in allergic airway inflammation. The above mechanism could be responsible for irritant and allergic reactions to pesticides.

The Agriculture Health Study by Hoppin demonstrated the relationship between pesticide application and chronic bronchitis among farmers (OR=1.83, 95% CI= 1.50, 2.24). This study which followed a cohort of 20,908 pesticide applicators was able to establish the role that similar groups of pesticides as the ones applied on tobacco have, in the development of chronic bronchitis[49]. One important finding was that AChE inhibitors (organochlorides and organophosphate) were predominantly associated with chronic bronchitis symptoms compared to other symptoms. While it was feasible to isolate the groups of pesticides in their study the farmers in our study had concurrent exposures to multiple pesticides some of which they could not remember. The higher odds of bronchitis in our study among pesticides exposed farmers suggest the synergistic or additive role of concurrent exposures.

This study showed a significant association between pesticide exposure and work-related upper airway symptoms. There was a positive but non-significant association between all proxies of pesticide exposure and work- related chest symptoms. Several studies have also reported similar associations while demonstrating the significant role that organophosphates had on those symptoms[97].

Furthermore, there was an association between duration of pesticide application in hours per day with some spirometry indices indicating airway limitation. Moderate to severe obstruction was strongest compared to isolated lower FEV1/FVC ratio. This is consistent with findings from several other studies which demonstrated a relationship between pesticide exposure and abnormal lung functions[42,97]. In these studies, AChE inhibitors including organophosphates, organochlorides and carbamates were shown to have a significant role in airway limitation.

Our participants reported extensive use of biomass fuel (87%), predominantly firewood (86%) almost daily. In the study done in urban Malawi there was a comparable proportion of biomass fuel use (85%), however, it was predominantly charcoal. Nearly half (44%) of the respondents indicated workplace exposure to biomass fuel and curing was reported as the source of this exposure. As much as 78% reported biomass fuel exposure through cooking (mainly at home). There were no differences in the type of fuel used for curing processes and cooking as they both use firewood. This might entail similar exposure characteristics between home users of firewood and those involved in curing at the workplace though dose of exposure might be different for those exposed in both home and workplace.

Biomass fuel use showed an increased significant association with work related nasal-ocular symptoms and protective against work related chest symptoms but did not demonstrate a substantive role in causing airway obstruction. The increased association with nasal-ocular symptoms might explain the acute effects of biomass fuel exposure which eventually leads to those individuals ceasing those tasks with time thereby demonstrating a protective effect for more chronic symptoms like chest symptoms. Biomass exposure at work showed an increased significant association with FEV_1<80% demonstrating a role in airflow limitation. This is contrary to a study in Malawi conducted in urban dwellers where biomass use at home did not show any significant association in causing airway obstruction[6]. Indoor air pollution through biomass fuel is a well-known cause of COPD despite our findings. In this study, it is evident that biomass fuel use was very common and involved nearly all participants making it unlikely to have power to show differential effects statistically among the participants who reported to have symptoms.

The findings of this study demonstrate the role of gender in occupational health. Males were employed for a relatively longer period than females. This might be due to the social set up in gender roles in the homes making females unable to sustain employment longer than males where males are considered bread winners and females being there to care for the homes[98]. Studies show that level of schooling is associated with personal health[99]. The fact that women had a relatively lower education level could easily make them more vulnerable to health risks in the workplace. Additionally, education level determines the ability to read and understand instructions including precautions against workplace hazards. Some respiratory outcomes showed differing pictures of association with gender. Males reported a higher prevalence of childhood asthma compared to females. Females reported a higher rate of eye symptoms and more women had an FEV_1 less than the lower limit of normal (LLN) than men. No other outcomes have shown a significant increased association with gender. Considering the relatively shorter period of employment among females and the higher rate of respiratory outcomes observed, it might explain the role of some gender specific vulnerabilities that disproportionately put females at an increased risk of respiratory outcomes in these occupational settings.

This study shows an increased risk of obstructive airway conditions among tobacco farmers in Malawi exposed to pesticides and nicotine. This study has employed the use of standardized outcome definitions and spirometry measurements to determine outcomes in this group of agricultural workers, enhancing the robustness of estimates generated and adding to an understanding of risk to respiratory health faced by tobacco farmers.

This study had several limitations. Firstly, the study design, being cross-sectional could not establish the causal relationship between the exposures and the outcomes. Secondly, the sample population being from one district and among flue cured tobacco farmers limits the generalizability of this study to the whole tobacco industry in Malawi which is dominated by burley tobacco. Thirdly, the convenient sampling method could subject it to selection bias with possibility of a healthy worker effect on our findings making us miss more serious cases of poor respiratory health. This would have the effect of underestimating the risk and attenuating the positive associations found. Fourthly, the use of questionnaire- based proxies of exposures and outcomes were subject to recall bias potentially leading to differential recall among the symptomatic cases compared to, asymptomatic individuals who could have significant levels of exposure.

In conclusion, this study has shown that tobacco farmers in Malawi have a higher prevalence of asthma and chronic bronchitis compared to farmers in other settings and the general population. Additionally, nicotine and pesticide exposures are key factors associated with obstructive lung diseases including work related upper and lower airway symptoms among the farmers with nicotine showing the strongest relationship in this regard.

This study which was aimed at investigating the risk factors associated with obstructive airway diseases among Malawian tobacco farmers has concluded that these farmers are at an increased risk of developing obstructive lung disease which is strongly associated with their exposure to nicotine and pesticides in the workplace.

Several recommendations are proposed to safeguard the health and safety of these tobacco farm workers against these commonly encountered hazards in the workplace.

Firstly, necessary legislation needs to be enacted or reviewed to include seasonal workers in tobacco estates as employees to be protected by the Occupational Safety, Health and Welfare Act (OSHWA) of 1997[100]. The current legislation does not recognize these estates as being workplaces governed by the particular act. According to the Malawi Occupational Health Profile of 2009[101] the informal sector constitutes 89% of the labor force and seasonal workers in tobacco estates fall under that majority category of workers who are not properly protected by the law. Legislation is a paramount driver of occupational health practice globally and any efforts to implement occupational health and safety would prove futile in the absence of proper legislation. The effectiveness of the existing legislation should be measured in its ability to promote the common good of the citizenry. In this instance having the legislation in place which cannot protect nearly 90% of the potential beneficiaries is a serious concern. While the OSHWA 1997 itself is lacking, the other necessary act is the Workers Compensation Act (WCA)[102]. This act ensures justice for those that become victims under the provisions of the OSHWA. It is noted that the current WCA does not schedule such common occupational respiratory diseases as Asthma, Rhinitis, COPD. This observation means that workers suffering from these conditions are likely to go unreported and not compensated eventually for their disability. It is also recommended that the WCA be reviewed to make it cover the Malawian workforce adequately.

Secondly, during this study, it was noted that tobacco estates do not follow strict safety measures of handling hazardous chemicals. For example, farms do not use recommended list of pesticides as published by the Tobacco Commission[26]; applicants do not use PPE adequately; other workers are not adequately protected from exposure during spraying times. The tobacco cultivation sector needs to enforce strict occupational hygiene principles for handling any hazardous substances including pesticides. There is a need for the proper practice of hierarchy of controls when dealing with the common hazards in these farms.

There is also a need to adopt an understanding that nicotine is a chemical hazard associated with serious reversible and non-reversible health effects and, therefore, exposure to it needs to be regulated with possible use of PPE for all workers handling tobacco as is the practice in other countries. Training is also necessary for all the workers to be conversant with some safety standards of practice in handling these workplace hazards.

Thirdly, due to the nature of these health effects it is necessary to institute a medical surveillance program for all tobacco workers in their workplaces. This would be the responsibility of the ministry of health, ministry of labor along with the Tobacco Commission. This is justified by the levels of toxicity of the chemicals that farmers are exposed to and the high prevalence of undetected health effects among them. Medical surveillance program will be an important tool for early detection of these health effects in this vulnerable population. Some of the important actions taken following such exercise would be: reducing exposure by switching or withdrawing affected employees from insulting hazards; treating the affected employees; rehabilitation; and compensation.

Fourthly, the regulatory authority for tobacco production, the Tobacco Commission, needs to consider health and safety compliance as one mandatory requirement for licensing tobacco producers in the country. Such a recommendation necessitates frequent inspections and audits among the farms by the authority to ensure compliance with the set standards. Heavy penalties need to be attached to noncompliance of such standards as the consequences constitute a violation of human rights.

Another issue to be considered is the implementation of workplace HIV/AIDS policy[103] in these workplaces. Considering the number of employees and the HIV burden at such workplaces deliberate efforts need to be put in place through employers and other partners to include these workers in HIV/AIDS information, education and communication. From the findings of this study it was evident that the prevalence was more than double compared to rural average in these workplaces signifying a very high concentration of the people living with HIV. These people need different kinds of support services for them to live a healthy and productive life. The HIV workplace policy of Malawi encourages workplace to design work in such a way that does not compromise the health and wellbeing of those infected. Other initiatives include special support for the employees who voluntarily disclose their status and zero discrimination at workplace on the basis of HIV status.

There are some recommendations for further research which would establish more evidence regarding health effects of tobacco cultivation. Some key areas that did not form the basis of data collected in this study and need further consideration include the following:

- Quantitative analysis of the particular exposures based on environmental and hygiene surveys;
- Pathophysiological mechanisms of nicotine and pesticides in causing obstructive diseases among tobacco farmers;
- Exploration of particular gender aspects associated with exposures in tobacco farmers.

REFERENCES

1. FAO. *Issues in the Global Tobacco Economy: Selected Case Studies.*; 2003.

2. Schmitt NM, Schmitt J, Kouimintzis DJ, Kirch W. Health risks in tobacco farm workers - A review of the literature. *J Public Health (Bangkok).* 2007;15(4):255-264. doi:10.1007/s10389-007-0122-4

3. Riquinho DL, Hennington EA. Health, environment and working conditions in tobacco cultivation: a review of the literature. *Cien Saude Colet.* 2012;17(6):1587-1600. doi:10.1590/S1413-81232012000600022

4. Kapatuka D. *Hard Work , Long Hours and Little Pay.*; 2009.

5. Gordon S, Graham S. Epidemiology of Respiratory Disease in Malawi. *Malawi Med J.* 2006;18(September):134-146.

6. Meghji J, Nadeau G, Davis KJ, et al. Noncommunicable lung disease in sub-Saharan Africa a community-based cross-sectional study of adults in urban Malawi. *Am J Respir Crit Care Med.* 2016;194(1):67-76. doi:10.1164/rccm.201509-1807OC

7. Lecours N, Almeida GEG, Abdallah JM, Novotny TE. Environmental health impacts of tobacco farming: a review of the literature. *Tob Control.* 2012;21(2):191-196. doi:10.1136/tobaccocontrol-2011-050318

8. Ngajilo D, Mbchb SA. Occupational allergy and asthma in tobacco farmers : a review of literature. *Curr Allergy Clin Immunol.* 2018;31(2):88-95.

9. TCCM. Tobacco Varieties. Tobacco Control Commission Publications. Malawi.

10. Arcury TA, Quandt SA, Arcury TA. Health and Social Impacts of Tobacco Production Health and Social Impacts of Tobacco Production. 2017;0813(April):71-81. doi:10.1300/J096v11n03

11. Kishi M, Hirschhorn N, Djajadisastra M, Satterlee LN, Strowman S, Dilts R. Relationship of pesticide spraying to signs and symptoms in Indonesian farmers. *Scand J Work Environ Heal.* 1995;21(2):124-133. doi:10.2307/40966340

12. Saleeon T, Siriwong W, Maldonado-pérez HL, Gregory M. The correlation between pesticide exposure and green tobacco sickness among Thai traditional tobacco farmers in Nan province. 2015;6(June):82-89.

13. Fiori N. Wheezing in tobacco farm workers in southern Brazil. *Am J Ind Med.* 2015;58(11):1217-1228.

14. Viegi G, Paggiaro PL, Begliomini E, Vaghetti E, Giuntini C. Respiratory effects of occupational exposure to tobacco dust. 1986:802-808.

15. Hang YZ, Ang JW, Ou JL. The Dose-Response Relationship between Pulmonary Function Injury and Cumulative Dose of Tobacco Dust Exposure among Tobacco Processing Workers. 2009;(168):164-168.

16. Etemadinejad S, Mohammadian M, Alizadeh-larimi A. Indian Journal of Medical Sciences pulmonary function in workers exposed to tobacco dust. 2009;63(12):543-548. doi:10.4103/0019-5359.59987

17. Oxford H. Review of Respirable Particle Size. 2013;(6).

18. Kirkhorn S. Agricultural Lung Diseases. *Environ Health Perspect*. 2000;108:705-712.

19. Schenker M. Exposures and health effects from inorganic agricultural dusts. *Environ Health Perspect*. 2000;108(SUPPL. 4):661-664.

20. Chloros D., Sichletidis L. b, Kyriazis G., Vlachogianni E., Kottakis I., Kakoura M. Respiratory effects in workers processing dried tobacco leaves. *Allergol Immunopathol (Madr)*. 2004;32(6):344-351. http://www.scopus.com/inward/record.url?eid=2-s2.0-14344265091&partnerID=40&md5=39d5d83bf22f168134ca236917ad36da.

21. Mishra A, Chaturvedi P, Datta S, Sinukumar S, Joshi P, Garg A. Harmful effects of nicotine. *Indian J Med Paediatr Oncol*. 2015;36(1):24-31. doi:10.4103/0971-5851.151771

22. Benowitz NL, Hukkanen J, Jacob P. Nicotine Psychopharmacology. *Handb Exp Pharmacol*. 2009;192(192):29-60. doi:10.1007/978-3-540-69248-5

23. CDC. Nicotine biomonitoring.

24. Onuki M; Yokoyama. Assessment of urinary cotinine as a marker of nicotine absorption from tobacco leaves: a study on tobacco farmers in Malaysia. *J Occup Health*. 2003;45(3):140-145.

25. Satora, L; Goszcz. Green tobacco sickness in Poland. *Pol Arch Med Wewn*. 2009;119(3):184-185.

26. Tobacco Control Commission. Pesticides Recommended for Use on Tobacco in Malawi 2017/18. 2017:1-8.

27. Jaga K, Dharmani C. Sources of exposure to and public health implications of organophosphate pesticides. 2003;14(3):171-185.

28. Ye M, Beach J, Martin JW, Senthilselvan A. Occupational pesticide exposures

and respiratory health. *Int J Environ Res Public Health*. 2013;10(12):6442-6471. doi:10.3390/ijerph10126442

29.   Kapka-skrzypczak L, Cyranka M, Skrzypczak M, Kruszewski M. Biomonitoring and biomarkers of organophosphate pesticides exposure – state of the art. 2011;18(2):294-303.

30.   Müller N, Faria X, Facchini LA, Fassa AG, Tomasi E. Pesticides and respiratory symptoms among farmers Agrotóxicos e sintomas respiratórios entre agricultores. *Rev Saúde Pública*. 2005;39(6):973-981. doi:/S0034-89102005000600016

31.   Arcury TA; Quandt SA; Predictors of incidence and prevalence of green tobacco sickness among latino farm workers in North Carolina. *J Epidemiol Community Heal*. 2001;55(11):818-824.

32.   Fassa AG, Faria NMX, Meucci RD. Green Tobacco Sickness Among Tobacco Farmers in Southern Brazil. *Am J Ind Med*. 2014:1-10. doi:10.1002/ajim.22307.

33.   Ballard TEJF. Green tobacco sickness: occupational nicotine poisoning in tobacco workers. *Arch Env Heal*. 1995;50(5):384-389.

34.   Curwin, BD; Hein, MJ; Sanderson. Nicotine exposure and decontamination on tobacco harvesters' hands. *Ann Occup Hyg*. 2005;49(5):407-413.

35.   Gosh, SK; Gokani VPJ. Protection against "green symptoms" from tobacco in Indian harvesters: a preliminary intervention study. *Arch Env Heal*. 1987;42(2):121-124.

36.   Lander F, Gravesen S. Respiratory disorders among tobacco workers. 2014;(November):500-502. doi:10.1136/oem.45.7.500

37.   Van Minh H, Giang KB, Bich NN, Huong NT. Tobacco farming in rural Vietnam: questionable economic gain but evident health risks. *BMC Public Health*. 2009;9:24-33. doi:10.1186/1471-2458-9-24

38.   Mustajbegovic J, Zuskin E, Schachter EN, Kern J, Luburic-Milas M, Pucarin J. Respiratory findings in tobacco workers. *Chest*. 2003;123(5):1740-1748. doi:10.1378/chest.123.5.1740

39.   Hoppin JA, Umbach DM, London SJ, Lynch CF, Alavanja MCR, Sandler DP. Pesticides associated with wheeze among commercial pesticide applicators in the agricultural health study. *Am J Epidemiol*. 2006;163(12):1129-1137. doi:10.1093/aje/kwj138

40.   Mwanga H, Jeebhay MF, Dalvie A. THE RELATIONSHIP BETWEEN

PESTICIDE METABOLITES AND ASTHMA OUTCOMES AMONG WOMEN FARM WORKERS. 2013.

41. Ndlovu V et al. Respiratory Allergy and Asthma associated with Pesticide Exposure amongst Women in Rural Western Cape. *Respir J Ind Medicne.* 2014:1331-1343.

42. Antonio H et al. Low Level of Exposure to Pesticides Leads to Lung Dysfunction in Occupationally Exposed Subjects. *Inhal Toxicol.* 2008;20(9):839-849.

43. Klintberg B, Berglund N, Lilja G, Wickman M, van Hage-Hamsten M. Fewer allergic respiratory disorders among farmers' children in a closed birth cohort from Sweden. *Eur Respir J.* 2001;17(6):1151-1157. doi:10.1183/09031936.01.00027301

44. Douwes J, Travier N, Huang K, et al. Lifelong farm exposure may strongly reduce the risk of asthma in adults. *Allergy Eur J Allergy Clin Immunol.* 2007;62(10):1158-1165. doi:10.1111/j.1398-9995.2007.01490.x

45. Alfvén T, Braun-Fahrländer C, Brunekreef B, et al. Allergic diseases and atopic sensitization in children related to farming and anthroposophic lifestyle - The PARSIFAL study. *Allergy Eur J Allergy Clin Immunol.* 2006;61(4):414-421. doi:10.1111/j.1398-9995.2005.00939.x

46. Mamane A, Baldi I, Tessier J, Raherison C, Bouvier G. Occupational exposure to pesticides and respiratory health. 2015:306-319. doi:10.1183/16000617.00006014

47. Ignacak A, Guzik T. The effect of chronic exposure to tobacco dust on the nasal mucosa The effect of chronic exposure is tobacco dust on nasal mucosa. *Allergy Asthma Immunol.* 2001;6(3):149-154.

48. Hoppin JA, Umbach DM, Long S, et al. Pesticides Are Associated with Allergic and Non-Allergic Wheeze among Male Farmers. *Environ Health Perspect.* 2016;(April):1-35. doi:10.1289/EHP315

49. Hoppin JA, Valcin M, Henneberger PK, et al. Pesticide Use And Chronic Bronchitis Among Farmers in The Agricultural Health Study. *Am J Ind Med.* 2010;50(12):969-979. doi:10.1002/ajim.20523.Pesticide

50. Muller N, Faria X, Fassa AG, Meucci RD, Fiori NS, Miranda VI. NeuroToxicology Occupational exposure to pesticides , nicotine and minor psychiatric disorders among tobacco farmers in southern Brazil.

Neurotoxicology. 2014;45:347-354. doi:10.1016/j.neuro.2014.05.002

51.   Blanc PD, Iribarren C, Trupin L, et al. Occupational exposures and the risk of COPD : dusty trades revisited. 2009:6-12. doi:10.1136/thx.2008.099390

52.   Esmaeil N, Gharagozloo M, Rezaei A, Grunig G. Dust events , pulmonary diseases and immune system. 2014;3(1):20-29.

53.   Schenker M et al. Inorganic Agricultural Dust Exposure Causes Pneumoconiosis among Farmworkers. *Proc Am Thorac Soc.* 2010;7:107-110. doi:10.1513/pats.200906-036RM

54.   Ramazzini C. 18/03/2016 Draft v1. 2016:1-13.

55.   Melbostad E, Eduard W, Magnus P, Wijnand E, Magnus P. Chronic bronchitis in farmers. *Scand J Work Environ Heal.* 1997;23(4):271-280. doi:10.5271/sjweh.220

56.   Osim EM. Lung function of Zimbabwean farm workers exposed to flu curing and stacking of tobacco leaves. *S Afr Med Journey.* 1998;88(9):1127-1131.

57.   Chen EY, Sun A, Chen C-S, Mintz AJ, Chin W-C. Nicotine alters mucin rheological properties. *Am J Physiol Lung Cell Mol Physiol.* 2014;307(2):L149-57. doi:10.1152/ajplung.00396.2012

58.   He F, Li B, Zhao Z, et al. The pro-proliferative effects of nicotine and its underlying mechanism on rat airway smooth muscle cells. *PLoS One.* 2014;9(4):1-14. doi:10.1371/journal.pone.0093508

59.   Eduard W, Douwes J, Omenaas E, Heederik D. Do farming exposures cause or prevent asthma? Results from a study of adult Norwegian farmers. *Thorax.* 2004;59(5):381-386. doi:10.1136/thx.2004.013326

60.   Stallones LBC. Pesticide poisoning and depressive symptoms among farm residents. *Ann Epidemiol.* 2002;12(6):389-394.

61.   McKnight RSH. Green tobacco sickness in children and adolescents. *Public Heal Rep.* 2005;120(6):602-605.

62.   Morris A, George MP, Crothers K, et al. HIV and chronic obstructive pulmonary disease: is it worse and why? *Proc Am Thorac Soc.* 2011;8(3):320-325. doi:10.1513/pats.201006-045WR

63.   Gingo MGM. Pulmonary function abnormalities in HIV-infected patients during the current antiretroviral therapy era. *Am J Crit Care Med.* 2010;182:790-796.

64.   Yearsley MDP. Correletion of HIV-1 detection and histology in AIDS-associated emphysema. *Diagn Mol Pathol.* 2005;14:48-52.

65. WHO. Tuberculosis and HIV. HIV/AIDS Topical information.

66. Friedland G. Tuberculosis and HIV Coinfection: Current State of Knowledge and Research Priorities. *J Infect Dis*. 2007;196:s1-s3.

67. Calvo M, Laguno M, Martinez M, Martinez E. Effects of tobacco smoking on HIV-infected individuals. *Aids Rev*. 2015;17(1):47-55. http://www.ncbi.nlm.nih.gov/pubmed/25427101.

68. Casaril M, Teixeira CDC, Mantovani VM, De A. Tobacco growing versus the health of tobacco growers. *Texto Context Enferm*. 2016;25(2):1-9.

69. Cai L, Wu X, Goyal A, et al. Patterns and socioeconomic influences of tobacco exposure in tobacco cultivating rural areas of Yunnan Province , China. *BMC Public Health*. 2012;12(1):1-8. doi:10.1186/1471-2458-12-842

70. WRI; *Pubmed World Resouces: A Guide to Global Environment*.; 1998.

71. Das I. Biomass cooking fuels and health outcomes for women in Malawi. *Ecohealth*. 2016;14:7-19.

72. Kurmi OP, Semple S, Devereux GS, et al. The effect of exposure to biomass smoke on respiratory symptoms in adult rural and urban Nepalese populations. *Environ Heal*. 2014;13(1):92. doi:10.1186/1476-069X-13-92

73. Guoping H et al. Risk of COPD from Exposure to Biomass Smoke: A Metaanalysis. *Chest*. 2010;138(1):20-31.

74. Smit RNVZ, Pai M, Yew WW, et al. Global lung health: the colliding epidemics of tuberculosis, tobacco smoking, HIV and COPD. 2010;35(1):27-33. doi:10.1183/09031936.00072909

75. Tobacco Control Commission. *Flue Cured Tobacco Farmers in Southern Malawi*.; 2017.

76. Adeloye D, Lee C, Papana A, Nair H, Sridhar D, Chan KY. Global and regional estimates of COPD prevalence : Systematic review and meta – analysis. 2015;5(2):1-17. doi:10.7189/jogh.05.020415

77. Sample Size Calculator. www.surveysystems.com. Published 2017.

78. Elam NE. Sample size calculation. 2005. http://www.depts.ttu.edu/afs/home/mgalyean/.

79. Miller MR, Hankinson J, Brusasco V, et al. Standardisation of spirometry. 2005;26(2):319-338. doi:10.1183/09031936.05.00034805

80. WHO. *Malawi STEPS NCD Risk Factor Survey 2017*.; 2017.

81. Lopes J, Dalke F, Müller M, Farianadia X. Alcohol consumption among

tobacco farmers : prevalence and associated factors. *Cience saude colet.* 2018;23(3):19-24.

82. MALAWI(NSO). *Malawi Demographic Health Survey 2016.*; 2017.

83. Crampin AC, Glynn JR, Ngwira BMM, et al. Trends and measurement of HIV prevalence in northern Malawi. *AIDS.* 2003;17(November 2002):1817-1825. doi:10.1097/01.aids.0000076278.54156.7e

84. Gislason T. Risk Factors for Chronic Obstructive Pulmonary Disease in a European Cohort of Young Adults. *Am J Respir Crit Care Med.* 2011;183(11):891-897. doi:10.1164/rccm.201007-1125OC

85. Nijs SB De, Venekamp LN, Bel EH. Adult-onset asthma : is it really different? 2013;22(127):44-52. doi:10.1183/09059180.00007112

86. Mirabelli MC, Hoppin JA, Chatterjee AB, et al. Job Activities and Respiratory Symptoms among farmworkers in North Carolina. *Arch Env Occup Heal.* 2012;66(3):178-182. doi:10.1080/19338244.2010.539637.Job

87. Ghosh SK, Parikh JR, Gokani VN, Rao MN, Kashyap SK. Studies on Occupational Health Problems in Agricultural Tobacco Workers *. 1980:113-117.

88. Osim EE, Musabayane C, Mufunda J. Lung function of Zimbabwean farm workers exposed to flue curing and stacking of tobacco leaves. 1998;(February 2014):1128-1131.

89. Hankinson JL. Values in a Multiethnic Sample of Adults. *Chest.* 2010;137(1):138-145. doi:10.1378/chest.09-0919

90. Ben H, Nour M, Attar E, Hadj K, Ben A. ScienceDirect The recent multi-ethnic global lung initiative 2012 (GLI 2012) reference values don 't reflect contemporary adult 's North African spirometry. *Respir Med.* 2013;107:2000-2008. doi:10.1016/j.rmed.2013.10.015

91. American Lung Association. Supplement: American Thoracic Society: Respiratory Health Hazards in Agriculture. *Am Thorac Soc.* 1998;158(5):1-76.

92. Mcbride JVS, Altman DG, Klein M, White W. Green tobacco sickness. *Tob Control.* 1998;7:294-298.

93. Senthilselvan A. Association of Asthma with Use of Pesticides: Results of a Cross-Sectional Survey of Farmers. *AJRCCM.* 1992;146(4).

94. Baldi I. Agricultural Exposure and Asthma Risk in the AGRICAN French Cohort. *Int J Hyg Environ Heal.* 2013.

95. Review M. Do Environmental Toxicants Contribute to Allergy and Asthma? *Altern Med Rev*. 2012;17(1):6-18.

96. Shaffo FC, Grodzki AC, Fryer AD, Lein XPJ. Mechanisms of organophosphorus pesticide toxicity in the context of airway hyperreactivity and asthma. 2018;315:L485-L501. doi:10.1152/ajplung.00211.2018

97. Chakraborty S. Chronic Exposure to Cholinesterase-Inhibiting Pesticides Adversely Affect Respiratory Health of Agricultural Workers in India. *J Occup Health*. 2009;51(6):488-497.

98. Kachiwanda SO. Gender disparity in the acquisition of literacy in sub-Saharan Africa : the case of Malawi. *J Humanit*. 2015;22:24-43.

99. Smith-greenaway E. Are literacy skills associated with young adults' health in africa? Evidence from malawi. *Soc Sci Med*. 2015;127:124-133. doi:10.1016/j.socscimed.2014.07.036.ARE

100. Malawi. *Occupational Safety, Health and Welfare Act Of Malawi, 1997.*; 1997.

101. Malawi. Malawi Country Profile on Occupational Safety And Health 2009. 2009.

102. Malawi. *Workers ' Compensation Act.*; 1999.

103. Malawi. *National HIV and AIDS Workplace Policy.*; 2010.

APPENDIX 1: RESEARCH ETHICS APPROVAL CERTIFICATE

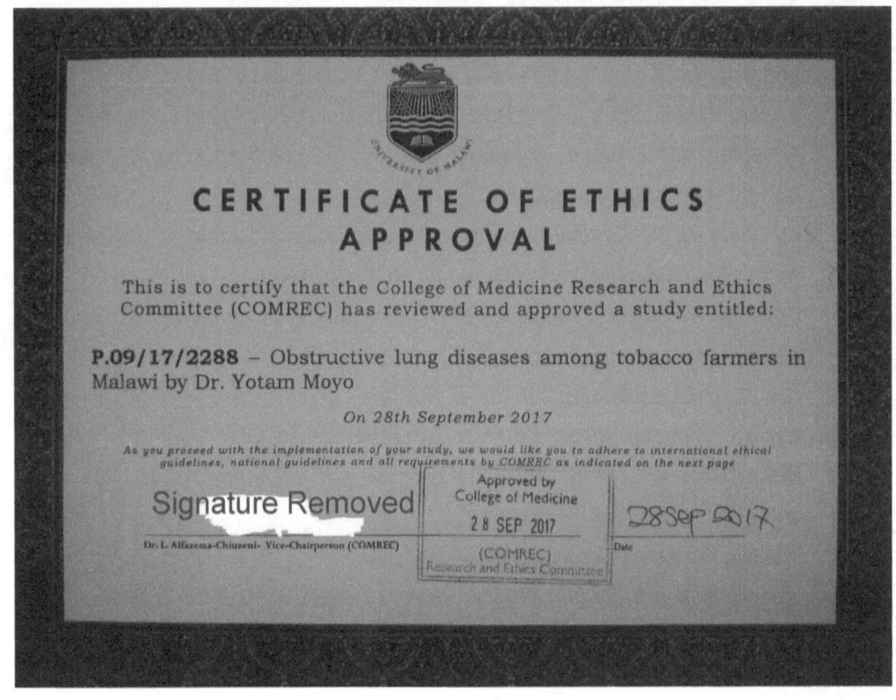

APPENDIX 2: PERMISSION FROM TOBACCO COMMISION

THE
TOBACCO CONTROL COMMISSION

P.O. Box 40045	P.O. Box 5080	P.O. Box 20321
Kanengo	LIMBE	Luwinga
LILONGWE 4	MALAWI	MZUZU 2
MALAWI		MALAWI
Tel : 01 712 777/01 712 305	Tel : 01 840 118	Tel : 01 320 947
Fax : 01 712 632/01 712 676	01 840 681	01 320 272
Email : tcclib@tccmw.co	Fax : 01 840 681	Fax : 01 320 832
Website : www.tccmw.co	Email: limbe@tccmw.com	Email: mzuzu@tccmw.com

3rd August 2017

Dr. Yotam Moyo

P. O. Box 1435

Blantyre

Dear Sir,

PERMISSION TO CONDUCT RESEARCH PROJECT AMONG MALAWIAN TOBACCO FARMERS

Reference is made to your letter dated 16th February 2017 requesting for permission to conduct a research among Malawian tobacco farmers. The Commission has no objection to your request.

I wish you all the best in your research and you are requested to appraise the Commission on the developments.

Regards

Signature Removed

David Luka

ACTING CHIEF EXECUTIVE OFFICER

APPENDIX 3: INFORMED CONSENT

UCT STUDY OF OBSTRUCTIVE LUNG DISEASES AMONG TOBACCO FARMERS IN MALAWI – 2017

ENGLISH CONSENT FORM

1. **Title of research project**

   A study of obstructive lung diseases among tobacco farmers in Malawi

2. **Purpose of the research**

   This research will form a basis for master's degree program and will also help to inform us about the extent of chronic lung diseases in Malawian tobacco farmers and possible contributors to such diseases. This information may help us to come up with proper interventions aimed at reducing the prevalence of such diseases.

3. **Description of the research project**

   If you agree to participate you will be asked to complete the following tests during working time:

   a) **Complete a questionnaire**

   A member of our study team will interview you in privacy to complete the questionnaire. You will be asked questions about respiratory diseases symptoms, current and previous employment history, risk factors related to potential harmful exposures (questions will cover environmental, occupational and personal factors).

   b) **Examination**

   A member of our study team will examine your body to measure blood pressure, weight, height, temperature as part of the process of gathering baseline health information

   c) **Spirometry Test and FeNO test**

   The team will examine the functioning of your lungs by conducting a spirometry test that requires you to forcefully exhale and blow through a portable machine held in your hands for a few seconds. They will also assess the response of your airway to allergens by asking you to blow exhaled air through another machine.

   d) **Urine test**

A urine test will be done to measure the presence of nicotine in your urine. A member of the study team will require a 50ml urine sample from you for that purpose. The urine samples will be stored and may be tested to look for the presence of other biological substances (biomarkers) at a later stage.

e) **Blood test**

Venous blood will be collected from you by trained personnel into two tubes and will be sent to a laboratory to check for an immune response to allergens as well as pesticides exposure. The blood samples will be stored and may be tested to look for the presence of other biological substances (biomarkers) at a later stage.

f) **HIV test**

You will be asked to provide documented results for your recent HIV test. If these are not available you will be asked to provide blood for an HIV test. This will be obtained from a fingerprick sample taken by a trained personnel and member of the research team. You will be asked whether you wish to be given your result. If you do wish to have your result, you will be referred to an independent agency for Voluntary, counselling and testing. This will include counseling and appropriate referral for further care depending on your test result. Your test result will be kept confidential and disclosed only to you. You have the right to refuse the HIV test but still enroll into the study.

4.   Confidentiality of information collected

Your name will not appear in any reports on this study. The records of spirometry, FeNO test, blood tests, and urine tests will be kept completely confidential and will be seen only by members of the study team.

5.   Risks and discomforts of the research

a) From the blood tests.
You will feel a single needle stick when the blood is taken. Sometimes a small bruise may occur from the needle stick, but this is minor and will heal quickly. The total amount of blood taken is quite small and your body will quickly replace it.

b) From Spirometry and FeNO
You may experience some discomfort due to the requirement to breathe out forcibly for three occasions otherwise it will be done within your capacity.

c) From urine test
You will submit this sample from your normal urine stream and we do not anticipate any discomfort to you during the collection of the urine sample.

d) From the questionnaire

There are no risks associated with the questionnaire and all information will be treated as confidential.

6.   **Expected benefits to you and to others**

You will be given a written copy of all your test results along with an explanation of what they mean, unless you tell us that you do not wish to receive this. You may wish to show these to your doctor if you are having any problems. These tests will help determine if you have any obstructive lung disease. Your participation will help to us understand the spectrum of respiratory health problems of tobacco farmers and may inform recommendations for better practices to safeguard health of workers engaged in tobacco farming.

7.   **Costs to you resulting from participation in the study**

The study is offered at no cost to you. In the event of an abnormal test result requiring further investigation or management you will be referred to a facility for further investigation and care

8.   **Voluntariness**

Your participation in this study is entirely voluntary and you are free to withdraw at any particular time and you shall not be penalized for doing so.

9.   **Contact person**.

You may contact the following person for answers to further questions about the research, your rights, or any injury you may feel is related to the study.

University of Cape Town Researchers:

Dr. Yotam Moyo, C/O Johns Hopkins Project, Queen Elizabeth Central Hospital Campus, P.O. Box 1131, Blantyre. Telephone No. (265) 999 329 438, Mobile No. (265) 888820011
Human Research Ethics Committee, E 53, Room 46, Old Main Building, Groote Schuur Hospital, Observatory Telephone: +27 21 406 6492

STUDY NO. _______________

10.   **Consent of the participant**

I have read the information given above, or it has been read to me. I understand the meaning of this information, Dr./Mr./Ms.

____

has offered to answer any questions concerning the study. By signing this form, I hereby consent to participate in the study. I also understand that I am free to withdraw from the study at any time without penalty.

11.   **Documentation of the consent**

One copy of this signed document will be kept together with our research records for this study. A copy of the information sheet about the study will be given to you to keep.

____

____
Print   Printed name of participant   Signature,   Mark,   or   Thumb

____

____
       Interviewer's name (Print)   Signature

DATE: ____________________

APPENDIX 4: GENERAL STUDY QUESTIONNAIRE

UCT OBSTRUCTIVE LUNG DISEASE AMONG MALAWIAN TOBACCO FARMERS - 2017/8

ENGLISH QUESTIONNAIRE
Note: Answer ALL questions. Insert a cross (X) where appropriate

Survey Number

Employer/Farm name:

Site or location:

Districts

A. DEMOGRAPHIC DATA

1. Surname

2. First name/s

3. Address

4. Work number

5. Date of birth: Day ___ Month ________ Year ___

6. Gender	
Male	1
Female	2

7. Years of schooling	
0	1
1-4	2
5-8	3
9-12	4

| | | >12 | 5 |

8. Home Language:		Chichewa	1
		Yao	2
		Lhomwe	3
		Sena	4
		Other	5

9. Are you a tenant or employee?		employee	1
		tenant	2
		other	3

10. Farm /estate size   Hectares [ ]

11. Amount of tobacco produced per season   Kg [ ]

12. Other crops grown on the farm

____

____

____

13. Employment duration (Years) [ ]

| 14. Work schedule/shift | _______________ __ | Day | 1 |
| | | Night | 2 |

15   Last work day?   Day ___   Month _______   Year ____

B. HEALTH PROBLEMS

Wheeze and tightness in the chest

| 1 | Have you ever had wheezing or whistling in your chest in the past? | Yes | 1 |
| | | No | 0 |

If YES, go on to Question 1.1
If NO, skip to Question 2

| 1.1 | If yes, when was the first time you had these symptoms? | Month _______   Year ____ |

| 1.2 | Have you had wheezing or whistling in your chest at any time in the **last 12 months**? | Yes | 1 |
| | | No | 0 |

If YES, go on to Question 1.2.1
If NO, skip to Question 3

1.2.1	Have you been short of breath when the wheezing noise was present?	Yes	1
		No	0
1.2.2	Have you had this wheezing or whistling when you did not have a cold or flu?	Yes	1
		No	0
2	Have you been woken up with a feeling of tightness in your chest at any time in the **last 12 months?**	Yes	1
		No	0

Shortness of breath

3	Have you had an attack of shortness of breath that came on during the daytime when you were at rest at any time in the **last 12 months?**	Yes	1
		No	0
4	Have you had an attack of shortness of breath that came on following running or exercise at any time in the **last 12 months?**	Yes	1
		No	0
5	Have you been woken by an attack of shortness of breath at any time in the **last 12 months?**	Yes	1
		No	0

Cough and phlegm from the chest

6	Have you been woken by an attack of coughing at any time in the **last 12 months?**	Yes	1
		No	0
7	Do you usually cough first thing in the morning?	Yes	1
		No	0
8	Do you usually cough during the rest of the day, or at night?	Yes	1
		No	0

If YES, go on to Question 8.1
If NO, skip to Question 9

8.1	Do you cough like this on most days/nights for as much as three or more months in each of the last two years?	Yes	1
		No	0
9	Do you usually bring up any phlegm from your chest first thing in the morning?	Yes	1
		No	0
10	Do you usually bring up any phlegm from your chest during the day, or at night?	Yes	1
		No	0

If YES, go on to Question 10.1

10.1	Do you bring up phlegm like this on most days/ nights for as much as three or more months in each of the last two years?	Yes	1	
		No	0	

Breathing

11	Do you ever have trouble with your breathing?	Yes	1
	If YES, go on to Question 11.1	No	0
	If NO, skip to Question 12		

11.1 Do you have this trouble:

Give all options at once

Insert a cross (X) next to one answer only

a) continuously so that your breathing is never quite right?	1
b) repeatedly, but it goes away completely between the times when it troubles you?	2
c) only rarely?	3

12	Are you disabled from walking by a condition other than heart or lung disease?	Yes	1
		No	0

If YES, state the condition and go on to Question 13
If NO, go to Question 12.1

12.1	Are you troubled by shortness of breath when hurrying on level ground or walking up a slight hill?	Yes	1
		No	0
	If YES, go on to Question 12.1.1		
	If NO, skip to Question 13		

12.1.1	Do you get short of breath walking with other people of your own age on level ground?	Yes	1
		No	0

12.1.2	Do you have to stop for breath when walking at your own pace on level ground?	Yes	1
		No	0

Asthma

13	Have you ever had asthma?	Yes	1
	If YES, go on to Question 13.1	No	0
	If NO, skip to Question 13.8		

13.1	If yes, was this confirmed by a doctor?	Yes	1
		No	0

13.2	How old were you when you were told you have		

asthma?

a) Only before you were 17 years old 1
b) Only at the age of 17 years or older 2
c) Both 3

13.3.1 How old were you when you had your first attack of asthma? ________ years old

13.3.2 How old were you when you had your most recent attack of asthma? ________ years old

13.4 Which months of the year do you usually have attacks of asthma?

13.4.1 January/February — Yes 1 / No 0

13.4.2 March/April — Yes 1 / No 0

13.4.3 May/June — Yes 1 / No 0

13.4.5 September/October — Yes 1 / No 0

13.4.6 November/December — Yes 1 / No 0

13.5 Have you had an attack of asthma in the last **12 months?** — Yes 1 / No 0

13.5.1 How often have you had an attack of asthma in

the **last 12 months?**

a) Every day   1
b) More than 2 times a week   2
c) More than 1 time per month   3
d) 3 to 12 times in the whole year   4
e) 1 to 2 times in the whole year   5

13.6   Are your chest symptoms caused by, or made worse by any of the following:

Answer all questions, insert a cross (X)

13.6.1   Contact with animals/pets   Yes 1   No 0

13.6.2   Grass or flowers   Yes 1   No 0

13.6.3   Heavy exercise   Yes 1   No 0

13.6.4   Breathing cold air   Yes 1   No 0

13.6.5   Dusts or sprays at work   Yes 1   No 0

13.6.6   Tobacco or other smoke   Yes 1   No 0

13.6.7   Change in the weather   Yes 1   No 0

13.7   Do your chest symptoms seem better or worse when you are away from work (for example, on weekends, off-shift and annual leave)?

a) Stay the same   1
b) Get better   2
c) Get worse   3

13.8   Does being at work ever make your chest tight   Yes 1

| | | | No | 0 |

or wheezy?

13.8.1 When did you first notice having problems with chest tightness or wheeze at work?   Month _______   Year ____

13.8.2 Is there anything that you work with **(specific activities in tobacco farming and related activities)** that causes you to have these chest symptoms?   Yes | 1   No | 0

13.8.3 What do you think is causing these symptoms?

____

13.9 Have you ever had to change or leave your work area, either temporarily or permanently, in this company or any other company because of any chest symptoms?   Yes | 1   No | 0

13.9.1 What type of job were you doing when this happened?

____

13.9.2 Was this job related to tobacco farming?   Yes | 1   No | 0

13.9.2.1 What area/section did you move to?

____

13.9.2.2 What job did you do there?

____

13.9.2.3 Did your symptoms improve when you changed jobs?   Yes | 1   No | 0

13.10. Have you ever worked in a job or jobs that exposed you to other than tobacco farming?   Yes | 1   No | 0

| 13.10.1 | What was or is this job? | ________________________ |
| | | (if current job write 'current job' and specify) |

| 13.10.2 | Before that? | ________________________ |

| 13.11 | Has there ever been **an instance** when you inhaled **a large amount** of vapour, gas or fumes in any of these jobs that resulted in you developing a tight chest, wheeze or cough? | Yes | 1 |
| | | No | 0 |

If YES, go on to Question 13.11.1.
If NO, skip to Question 13.12

| 13.11.1 | What was or is this job? | ________________________ |
| | | (if current job write 'current job' and specify) |

| 13.12 | Are you using any medicines, including inhalers/ pumps, nebulizers, syrups or tablets, for asthma or breathing problems? | Yes | 1 |
| | | No | 0 |

If YES, go on to Question 13.12.1, showing examples of each. If NO, skip to question 13.13

13.12.1	Which medicines?	________________________
		________________________
		________________________

| 13.12.2 | Do you take these medicines every day even when you do not have any trouble breathing? | Yes | 1 |
| | | No | 0 |

| 13.13 | Have you ever been treated for any of the following: | | |

Answer all questions

13.13.1	Repeated chest infections as a child	Yes	1
		No	0
		Unknown	2

13.13.2	Tuberculosis (TB)	Yes	1
		No	0
		Unknown	2

| 13.13.3 | Chronic bronchitis | Yes | 1 |
| | | No | 0 |

| | | Unknown | 2 |

13.13.4	HIV Status	Positive	1
	please verify with health passport	Negative	0
	otherwise, offer provider initiated testing	Unknown	2

<u>Nose and eye symptoms</u>

| 14 | Have you ever had any nose or eye problems or allergies such as allergic rhinitis ? | Yes | 1 |
| | | No | 0 |

If YES, go on to Question 14.1
Answer all questions
If NO, skip to Question 14.4

| 14.1 | How old were you when you first noticed these symptoms? | Years old | |

| 14.2 | During the past 12 months have you had **two or more** episodes of: | | |

| 14.2.1 | Sneezy, itchy or runny nose when you did not have a cold or flu? | Yes | 1 |
| | | No | 0 |

| 14.2.2 | Red, itchy or watery eyes | Yes | 1 |
| | | No | 0 |

| 14.2.3 | Do you usually have the nose or eye symptoms at any particular time of the year? | Yes | 1 |
| | | No | 0 |

14.2.3.1   If YES, which is the **worst** season?

<u>Give all options at once</u>
Insert a cross (X) next to ONE answer only

a) Winter	1
b) Summer	2
c) Spring	3
d) Autumn	4

If YES to any of question 14.2, go on to Question 14.3
If NO, skip to Question 14.4

14.3   Do your nose or eye symptoms seem better or

worse when you are away from work (for example, on
weekends, off-shift and annual leave?)

*__Give all
options at
once__*

Insert a cross (X) next to ONE answer only

a) Stay the same   1
b) Get better   2
c) Get worse   3

14.4   Does being at work ever cause you to have sneezy/   Yes   1
itchy/runny nose or red/itchy/watery eyes?   No   0

*If YES to any one of the above, go on to
Question 14.4.1*

If NO, skip to Question 14.6

14.4.1   Since when have you been having these
symptoms at work?   Month _________   Year _____

14.4.2   Is there anything that you work with **(e.g. "fresh"vs**   Yes   1
"dry" tobacco, **dust, pesticides)** or any other   No   0
substance that causes you to have these symptoms?

If YES, go on to Question 14.4.3

If NO, skip to Question 14.5

14.4.3   What do you think is causing these symptoms?

____

14.5   Are you using any medicines, including nose   Yes   1
sprays, drops, tablets or injections, for your nose or eye   No   0
symptoms at present?

If YES, go on to Question 14.5.1

If NO, go on to Question 14.6

*__Present a chart with different
allergy medicines__*
*(N.B. a worker might show you his/her
medicines).*

14.5.1   Which medicines?

____

____

14.6   Did you have hay fever (itchy or watery eyes/nose)   Yes   1
as a child?   No   0

GREEN TOBACCO SICKNESS SYMPTOMS

15   Have you ever had any of the following symptoms after coming into contact with tobacco leaves?

a) Headache	1
b) Dizziness	2
c) Nausea	3
d) Vomiting	4

15.1 How soon after work did you get the symptoms?

a) same day	1
b) day after	2
c) 2 days after	3
d) 3 days after	4
e) a week or more later	5

15.2 When did you have your most

recent attack of symptoms?   ________ years
    _   old

15.3 During which farm activities do you usually have
the symptoms in (15) above

15.3.1 Sowing   Yes 1 / No 0

15.3.2 Transplanting   Yes 1 / No 0

15.3.3 Harvesting   Yes 1 / No 0

15.3.4 Curing   Yes 1 / No 0

15.3.5 Other   Yes 1 / No 0

Specify ________________________

15.4 Have you had any of the reported symptoms in (15) in the last **12 months?**   Yes 1 / No 0

15.4.1	How many episodes of GTS symptoms have you had in the **last 12 months?**		

Give all options at once
Insert a cross (X) next to one answer only

a) None	0
b) One	1
c) Two	2
d) Three	3
e) Four or more	4

15.5 Are your symptoms caused by, or made
 worse by any of the following:

Answer all questions, insert a cross (X)

| 15.5.1 | harvesting tobacco | Yes | 1 |
| | | No | 0 |

| 15.5.2 | stacking | Yes | 1 |
| | | No | 0 |

| 15.5.3 | dust | Yes | 1 |
| | | No | 0 |

| 15.5.4 | curing tobacco | Yes | 1 |
| | | No | 0 |

| 15.5.5 | pesticde sprays at work | Yes | 1 |
| | | No | 0 |

| 15.5.6 | Tobacco or other smoke | Yes | 1 |
| | | No | 0 |

| 15.5.7 | Change in the weather | Yes | 1 |
| | | No | 0 |

15.6 Do your symptoms seem better or worse
when you are away from work (for example, on
weekends, off-shift and annual leave)?

Give all options at once
Insert a cross (X) next to ONE answer only

a) Stay the same	1
b) Get better	2

| | c) Get worse | | 3 |

| 15.7.1 | Is there anything that you work with **(specific activities in tobacco production facilities) that** causes you to have these symptoms? | Yes
No | 1
0 |

If YES, go on to Question 13.8.3
If NO, skip to Question 13.9

| 15.7.2 | What do you think is causing these symptoms? |

____

| 15.8 | Have you ever had to change or leave your work area, either temporarily or permanently, in this company or any other company because of any chest symptoms? | Yes
No | 1
0 |

If YES, go on to Question 13.9.1
If NO, skip to Question 13.10

| 15.9.1 | What type of job were you doing when this happened? |

| 15.9.2 | Was this job in this company? | Yes
No | 1
0 |

If YES, go on to Question 13.9.2.1
If NO, skip to Question 13.10

| 15.9.2.1 | What area/section did you move to? |

____

| 15.9.2.2 | What job did you do there? |

____

| 15.9.2.3 | Did your symptoms improve when you changed jobs? | Yes
No | 1
0 |

C. ALCOHOL AND DRUG USE

| 16.1 | Do you drink alcohol or did you drink before?
If no, proceed to 16.2 | Yes
No | 1
0 |

| 16.1.1 | Have you ever felt that you should drink less alcohol? | Yes
No | 1
0 |

| 16.1.2 | Have people ever angered you by criticizing your drinking habits? | Yes | 1 |
| | | No | 0 |

| 16.1.3 | Have you ever felt guilty or bad because you drink alcohol? | Yes | 1 |
| | | No | 0 |

| 16.1.4 | Have you ever had a drink early in the morning to make you feel better? | Yes | 1 |
| | | No | 0 |

16.2 — Have you ever smoked tobacco (cigarettes or pipe) for as long as a year?   Yes **1** / No **0**

('Yes' means at least 20 packs of cigarettes or 30 grams of tobacco in a lifetime or at least one cigarette per day for one year)

If no go to section D

16.2.1 — How old were you when you started smoking?   Age in Years ☐

16.2.2 — Do you smoke currently?   Yes **1** / No **0**

('Yes' means smoking tobacco in the last month or more)

16.2.3 — If no, how old were you when you stopped smoking?   Age in years ☐

16.2.3 — How much do/did you now smoke on average?

16.2.3.1 — Number of cigarettes per day ☐

16.2.3.2 — Pipe tobacco in grams/week ☐

16.2.4 — Do you or did you inhale the smoke?   Yes **1** / No **0**

16.3 — Have you been regularly exposed to tobacco smoke from other people smoking cigarettes or pipe in the **last 12 months?**   Yes **1** / No **0**

('Regularly' means on most days or nights)

16.4 — Do you take drugs or have taken drugs before?   Yes **1** / No **0**

If YES, please state for how many years ☐

D. FARM ACTIVITIES INVOLVED

1   Area/section _______________________ ☐

2	Job Title		

Get a short description of the job

____

____

____

____

3	Permanent/casual/tenant:	_______________

4	How long have you worked in this job?	Years		
		Months		

5	What types of tobacco do you work with?

please tick all that apply

a) Burley	1
b) Flue cured	2
c) Northern Division Dark fired (NDDF)	3
d) Southern Division Fired (SDF)	4
g) Other	5

Specify: _______________________________________

6	Do you ever do other farm tasks during your shift on	Yes	1
	a regular basis (almost every day)?	No	0

If **Yes**, which jobs?

____

____

7	Does your job involve these activities?	Yes	1

tick all that apply

		No	0

If YES, continue with 3.5.1 (one or more), If NO go to 3.5.2

a) Tilling	1
b) Spraying	2
c) Harvesting	3
d) Stacking	4
e) Curing	5
f) Sorting	6
g) Planting/transplanting	7
h) Sowing	8
i) Weeding	9
l) Transport	10

m) Administration	11
n) General cleaning	12
o) Cleaning equipment	13
p) Cleaning Personal Protective Equipment	14
q) Other	15

Specify: ____

7.1 How much dust would you say your current job produces:

Give all options at once

Insert a cross (X) next to ONE answer only

a) No dust	0
b) A little	1
c) A medium amount	2
d) A lot	3

7.1.1 How far do you work from the source of the dust?

Give all options at once

Insert a cross (X) next to ONE answer only

a) Right next to the source	1
b) About 1-2 metres away	2
c) More than 3 metres away	3
d) Does not apply	4

EXPOSURE TO PESTICIDES AT WORK

7.2 Does your work involve application (spray/mix) of pesticides _______________________________ Yes 1

_______________________________ No 0

7.2.1 If YES which pesticides do you use _______________________________

____

____

____

7.2.2 When last did you apply pesticides? _______________ Month _______ Year ____

7.2.3 How many months a year do you apply pesticides?

7.2.4	How many days per month do you apply pesticides in the spraying months?		
7.2.5	Total number of days per year		
7.2.6	How many hours per day do you work with pesticides?		
7.2.7	Do you do other field work while others spray pesticide?	Yes	1
		No	0
7.2.7.1	If yes, how many times per year?		

ENVIRONMENTAL PESTICIDES EXPPOSURE

7.3	Do you come into come into contact with pesticides outside the house while spraying occurs?	Yes	1
		No	0
7.3.1.	Does the pesticide spraying come into the house?	Yes	1
		No	0
7.3.2	Do you go into in the fields soon after spraying or come into contact with sprayed surfaces?	Yes	1
		No	0

HOME PESTICIDES EXPOSURE

7.4	Do you use pesticides at home	Yes	1

| | (spray/mix) of pesticides | | No | 0 |

| 7.4.1 | If YES which pesticides do you use | ______________________________ |

____

____

____

____

| 7.4.2 | When last did you use home pesticides? | ____________________ | Month _______ | Year ____ |

EXPOSURE TO BIOMASS FUEL

| 8.1 | Are you exposed to smoke from open fires used for cooking, heating, or curing purposes? | | Yes | 1 |
| | | | No | 0 |

| 8.1.1. | What is the source of this particular smoke? *(tick all that apply)* | | | |

firewood		1
charcoal		2
coal		3
other (please specify)		4

| 8.1.2 | If YES where do you come into contact with environmental smoke? | home | 1 |
| | | work | 2 |

8.1.3	What tasks expose you to smoke? Tick all that apply		
	cooking	1
	curing tobacco	2

| | smoking | 3 |
| | other | 4 |

| 8.1.4 | When last did you work/stay in smoky environment? | Month ____ | Year ____ |

| 8.1.5 | How many months a year do you work/stay in smoky environment? | |

| 8.1.6 | How many days per month do you work/stay in smoky environment? | |

| 8.1.7 | Total number of days per year | |

| 8.1.8 | How many hours per day do you work/stay in smoky environment? | |

Use of Personal Protective Equipment

| 9.1 | Do you use any personal protective equipment on a regular basis (almost every day) while doing your job? | Yes | 1 |
| | | No | 0 |

If NO, skip to Question 9.4

9.1.1 During which of the following do you were PPE? *(Tick all that apply)*

a) Tilling	1
b) Spraying	2
c) Harvesting	3
d) Stacking	4
e) Curing	5
f) Sorting	6

g) Planting/transplanting	7
h) Sowing	8
i) Weeding	9
l) Transport	10
m) Administration	11
n) General cleaning	12
o) Cleaning equipment	13
p) Cleaning Personal Protective Equipment	14
q) Other	15

Specify: _______________________________________

9.2.1 Which of the following personal protective equipment do you use on a **regular** basis (almost every day while working)?

9.2.1.1 Goggles:

Yes | 1
No | 0

9.2.1.2 Gloves:

Yes | 1
No | 0

9.2.1.3 Mask:

Yes | 1
No | 0

9.2.1.4 Work suite

Yes | 1
No | 0

9.2.1.5 Other:

Yes | 1
No | 0

Specify: _______________________________________

If NO to all of the previous questions, skip to Question 9.4

9.2.2 How long have you been wearing the personal protective equipment on a regular basis (almost every day) while working?
(0= 0 , 1=up to 1 year, 2= 2-3 years, 3= >3 years)

9.2.2.1 Goggles

9.2.2.2 Gloves:

9.2.2.3 Mask:

9.2.2.4	Aprons:		

9.2.2.5	Other:		

9.3	Is PPE provided free of charge?	Yes	1
		No	0

9.4	Do you have wash rooms to bath after applications	Yes	1
		No	0

	Do you have hand washing facilities at work to wash hands after work?	Yes	1
		No	0

Previous jobs in present company

10	Before doing this job at this company, did you do a different job here?	Yes	1
		No	0

If NO, skip to question 11
If YES, continue with question 10.1

10.1   What other jobs did you do here?

Start with the first job and work forward, getting a one-line description of each job. If casual worker, denote each period of employment as a separate job. For continuous years of seasonal work consider as one job (provided no broken years' service)

Job 1

10.1.1	Area/section		

10.1.2	Job Title		

Get a short description of the job

10.1.3	Permanent/casual/tenant:	

10.1.4	How long did you work in this job?	Years	
		Months	

10.1.5	In which area were you working?	
	a) Tilling	1
	b) Spraying	2
	c) Harvesting	3
	d) Stacking	4
	e) Curing	5
	f) Sorting	6
	g) Planting/transplanting	7
	h) Sowing	8
	i) Weeding	9
	j) Cleaning	10
	l) Transport	11
	m) Administration	12
	n) Other	13

Specify: ________________________________

10.1.7 How much dust would you say your previous job produced:

Give all options at once

Insert a cross (X) next to ONE answer only

a) No dust	0
b) A little	1
c) A medium amount	2
d) A lot	3

10.1.8 Did your job involve handling pesticides?   Yes | 1

Give all options at once

If YES, continue with 4.1.8 (one or more), If NO go to 4.1.9   No | 0

10.1.7. How much contact with pesticides did you have in your previous job?

Give all options at once

Insert a cross (X) next to ONE answer only

a) None	0
b) A little	1
c) A medium amount	2
d) A lot	3

10.1.7 How much contact with tobacco leaves did you have in your previous job?

Give all options at once

Insert a cross (X) next to ONE answer only

a) None	0
b) A little	1

c) A medium amount		2
d) A lot		3

10.1.7 How much contact with smoke did you have in your previous job?

a) None		0
b) A little		1
c) A medium amount		2
d) A lot		3

10.1.10 Did you use any personal protective equipment on a regular basis (almost every day) while doing your job?

Yes	1
No	0

If NO, skip to Question 4.2.1
If YES, continue with Question 4.1.10

10.1.10.1-5 Which of the following personal protective equipment did you use on a regular basis (almost every day)?

10.1.10.1 Goggles:

10.1.10.2 Gloves:

10.1.10.3 Mask:

10.1.10.4 Aprons:

10.1.10.5 Other:

If NO to all of the previous questions, skip to Question 4.2.1
If YES to any one of the above questions, continue with Question 4.1.11

10.1.11 How long have you been wearing the personal protective equipment on a regular basis (almost every day) while working?
(0= 0 , 1=up to 1 year, 2= 2-3 years, 3= >3 years)

10.1.11.1 Goggles

10.1.11.2	Gloves:	☐
10.1.11.3	Mask:	☐
10.1.11.4	Aprons:	☐
10.1.11.5	Other:	☐

Job 2

| 10.2.1 | Area/section | ☐☐ |
| 10.2.2 | Job Title | ☐☐ |

Get a short description of the job

____

____

____

____

| 10.2.3 | Permanent/casual/tenant: | _____________ |

10.2.4   How long did you work in this job?   Years ☐☐   Months ☐☐

10.2.5   In which area were you working?
a) Tilling
b) Spraying
c) Harvesting
d) Stacking
e) Curing
f) Sorting
g) Planting/transplanting
h) Sowing
i) Weeding
j) Cleaning
l) Transport
m) Administration
n) Other
Specify: _____________________________

10.2.7   How much dust would you say your previous job produced:

a) No dust	0
b) A little	1
c) A medium amount	2
d) A lot	3

10.2.8 Did your job involve handling pesticides? Yes 1 No 0

10.2.7 How much contact with pesticides did you have in your previous job?

a) None	0
b) A little	1
c) A medium amount	2
d) A lot	3

10.2.7 How much contact with tobacco leaves did you have in your previous job?

a) None	0
b) A little	1
c) A medium amount	2
d) A lot	3

10.2.7 How much contact with smoke did you have in your previous job?

a) None	0
b) A little	1
c) A medium amount	2
d) A lot	3

10.2.10 Did you use any personal protective equipment on a regular basis (almost every day) while doing your job? Yes 1 No 0

| 10.2.10.1-5 | Which of the following personal protective equipment did you use on a regular basis (almost every day)? | |

| 10.2.10.1. | Goggles: | ☐ |

| 10.2.10.2 | Gloves: | ☐ |

| 10.2.10.3 | Mask: | ☐ |

| 10.2.10.4 | Aprons: | ☐ |

| 10.2.10.5 | Other: | ☐ |

If NO to all of the previous questions, skip to Question 4.2.1
If YES to any one of the above questions, continue with
Question 4.1.11

| 10.2.11 | How long have you been wearing the personal protective equipment on a regular basis (almost every day) while working? **(0= 0 , 1=up to 1 year, 2= 2-3 years, 3= >3 years)** | |

| 10.2.11.1 | Goggles | ☐ |

| 10.2.11.2 | Gloves: | ☐ |

| 10.2.11.3 | Mask: | ☐ |

| 10.2.11.4 | Aprons: | ☐ |

| 10.2.11.5 | Other: | ☐ |

Previous work experience

| 11 | Name all the previous workplaces that you have worked in, when not working in this company or before coming to work in this company: ***Start with the most recent job and work backwards*** | |

Name of Company	What did the company make?	Job title (what did you do?)	Date started (year)	Date ended (year)	Total years

THANK YOU FOR ANSWERING THE QUESTIONNAIRE

Interviewer's name: ________________________________

Date of interview: Day ___   Month _______   Year ____

UCT STUDY OF OBSTRUCTIVE LUNG DISEASES AMONG TOBACCO FARMERS IN MALAWI – 2017/2018

LFT PRE-TEST DATA COLLECTION SHEET

Survey Number   ___________________

6. Date of interview:

Day____Month_________Year______

B.HEALTH PROBLEMS
Recent chest infections
1. Have you had the flu, sinusitis or a chest infection in the past 3 weeks?

Yes	(1)
No	(2)

2. Are you being treated for Tuberculosis (TB)?

Yes	(1)
No	(2)

2.1 If yes, for how long?   ________months   ________weeks

If YES, to question no 2, indicate to person that the tests will not be done today. Schedule another appointment in three months since the start of TB medication. If the person has already had three months of treatment, proceed with the rest of the screening questions and the post-bronchodilator test.

9. Have you had asthma in the past?

Yes	(1)
No	(2)

9.1 Do you have asthma now?

Yes	(1)
No	(2)

. Have you had any
of the following
symptoms in the
past 12 months?

   (at night, with exercise, exposure to cold air, viral infections, work exposures)

a)   chest tightness
b)   shortness of breath
c)   wheezing or whistling in your chest
d)   dry cough

12. Do you currently have any of these symptoms?

	Yes	(1)
	No	(2)

12.1 If Yes, which ones?
a)   chest tightness
b)   shortness of breath
c)   wheezing or whistling in your chest
d)   dry cough

3. Have you had a heart attack or stroke in the last month?

	Yes	(1)
	No	(2)

4. Do you have epilepsy?

	Yes	(1)
	No	(2)

5. Have you had an operation in the last 12 months?

	Yes	(1)
	No	(2)

If **YES** to any of the above **Q3-5**, indicate to the person that the lung function tests will not be done. If NO, proceed with the rest of the screening questions

6.For women:

6.1 Are you Pregnant?

	Yes	(1)
	No	(2)

6.2 Are you Breastfeeding?

	Yes	(1)
	No	(2)

If **Pregnant**, indicate to the person that the **Lung Function Test will not be done** today

---

If **Breastfeeding**, proceed with Lung Function Test with Post-Bronchodilator. Proceed with the rest of the screening questions.

C. MEDICATION USAGE (show booklet)

1. Are you taking any medicine/s from a doctor or clinic at the moment for asthma, and or hayfever?

Yes	(1)
No	(2)

1.1 If yes, what are you taking and when last did you take them?

Names   No. of hours since last dose

_______________________   _______________

_______________   _______________   _______________

_______________   _______________   _______________

2. Are you taking any medicine/s from a doctor or clinic at the moment for any heart condition, or your eyes?

Yes	(1)
No	(2)

If short-acting beta-2-agonist or anti-cholinergic inhalers used in the **last 4** hours or long-acting MDI or theophylline used in **last 8** hours, reschedule spirometry and counsel accordingly.

D. RECENT FOOD INTAKE

1. Did you drink coffee, tea or coca-cola in the last 6 hours?

Yes	(1)
No	(2)

2. Did you have anything to eat or drink in the last hour?

Yes	(1)
No	(2)

3. Have you smoked in the last hour?

Yes	(1)
No	(2)

If YES to Question 2 or 3, reschedule test for at least 1 hour later the same day or another date.

APPENDIX 6: LFT DATA SHEET

UCT STUDY OF OBSTRUCTIVE LUNG DISEASES AMONG TOBACCO FARMERS IN MALAWI – 2017

LUNG FUNCTION TESTS DATA COLLECTION SHEET

CARD 1

Record Number	1-3
Work number	4-9

Date   □□□ | □ □ | □□   10-15

DAY   MONTH   YEAR

1. Participant's blood pressure   □□□   systolic

□□□   diastolic

YEARS

2. Participant's age   □□   16-17

MALE   FEMALE

3. Participant's gender   □ □   18

CENTIMETRES

4.1 Participant's height   □□□   19-21

KILOGRAMS

4.2 Participant's weight   □□□   22-24

5. When did you last work in the farm?   Date   □□ □□ □□   25-30

<u>BASELINE SPIROMETRY</u>

6. **PREDICTED FEV$_1$**   □ □□   31-33

7. **INITIAL FEV$_1$ and FVC**
(up to 8 attempts)

	FEV$_1$	FVC	
1	□ □□	□ □□	34-39
2	□ □□	□ □□	40-45
3	□ □□	□ □□	46-51
4	□ □□	□ □□	52-57
5	□ □□	□ □□	58-63

7.1 Number of rejected attempts   □   64

8. **Best INITIAL FEV$_1$ as % of predicted FEV$_1$**   □□□   65-67

(divide best results from No. 7 by results from No. 6)

BRONCHODILATOR CHALLENGE ONLY

9. **FEV$_1$ and FVC**

FEV$_1$ FVC

9.1 Record Best two technically satisfactory   □ □□   □ □□   68-73
Manoeuvres (up to 8 attempts)   □ □□   □ □□   74-79

9.2 Number of rejected attempts   □   80

CARD 2

10. **Best POST-BRONCHODILATOR FEV$_1$ as % of initial FEV$_1$**   □□□   1-3

(divide best results from No. 9 by best results from No. 7)

11. General comments:

____

____

---

12. Technologist initial's _________________   □ 4

13. Room temperature: _______________   □□ 5-6
    (degrees celcius)

                                                    NO   YES
14 Lung function record appended   □   □   7